Perry Romanowski and the
THEBEAUTYBRAINS.COM

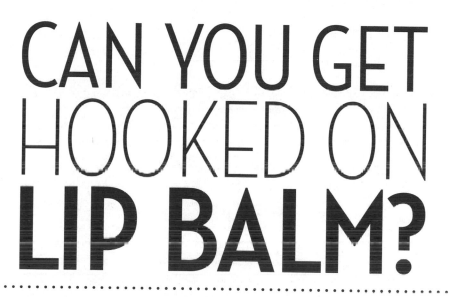

# CAN YOU GET HOOKED ON LIP BALM?

Top Cosmetic Scientists Answer Your
Questions about the Lotions, Potions and
Other Beauty Products You Use Every Day

To Beauty Brainiacs everywhere—
you can be beautiful *and* brainy

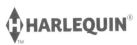

**CAN YOU GET HOOKED ON LIP BALM?**
ISBN-13: 978-0-373-89234-1
© 2011 by Brains Publishing

The opinions expressed here are those of the author and not necessarily those of the publisher. The advice in this book is intended only as an informative resource guide to help you make informed decisions; it is not meant to replace the advice of a physician or to serve as a guide to self-treatment. Always seek competent medical help for any health condition or if there is any question about the appropriateness of a product, procedure or health recommendation.

Library of Congress Cataloging-in-Publication Data
Romanowski, Perry, 1969—
    Can you get hooked on lip balm? : top cosmetic scientists answer your questions about
       the lotions, potions and other beauty products you use every day /
       Perry Romanowski and the creators of TheBeautyBrains.com.
       p. cm.
    Includes bibliographical references and index.
    ISBN 978-0-373-89234-1 (trade pbk.)
    1. Cosmetics—Popular works. I. TheBeautyBrains.com. II. Title.
    RA778.R615 2011
    646.7'2—dc22
    2010044199

www.eHarlequin.com

**Printed in U.S.A.**

# CONTENTS

## PART I    HAIR

**PART III**    **MAKEUP**

:::

## WHO ARE THE BEAUTY BRAINS?

The Beauty Brains are a group of cosmetic scientists who understand what the chemicals used in cosmetics really do, how products are tested, and what all the advertising means. They have no cosmetics to sell so you can be sure that the information provided is the most unbiased beauty advice available.

### LEFT BRAIN

The most hard-core skeptical scientist of all the Beauty Brains, the Left Brain peruses the world of science to bring you the latest developments and explain how they might apply to the cosmetic world.

### RIGHT BRAIN

Still scientific, but a bit less militant, the Right Brain has a good eye for the humorous—and human interest—side of science. The Right Brain is particularly skilled in interpreting advertising claims.

### SARAH BELLUM

Sarah works behind the scenes researching questions, reviewing the latest beauty technology and acting as the Beauty Brains' guinea pig.

# WHAT'S THE PURPOSE OF THE BEAUTY BRAINS?

There are literally *thousands* of cosmetic products and companies constantly bombarding you with confusing, and sometimes false, claims. The Beauty Brains was started in 2006 to help women understand the real science behind the beauty products they use every day. We have taken questions from people around the world about all beauty topics, including hair care, skin care, makeup and even cosmetic surgery.

We're here to help you cut through the confusing, misleading and sometimes false information with which the beauty companies bombard you. Our goal is to explain cosmetic science to you in a way that's entertaining and easy to understand. We believe the more information you have, the better you'll be able to find products that you like at a price you can afford. So you can listen to the advertising, or advice from a friend, or what your stylist tells you. But if you really want to understand cosmetic products in an unbiased, scientific way, you need the Beauty Brains.

In this book we've collected our best questions and answers to make learning about cosmetic science easy and entertaining. By giving you honest, unbiased information, the Beauty Brains can help you become a smarter shopper so you'll be able to get the products you like at prices you can afford.

# PART I

# HAIR

# 1 HAIR PRODUCTS FROM SALONS TO STORES

Stylists love to push products but is it really the best idea to buy them? In this chapter, you'll learn the truth about whether salon brands are really exclusive to salons, the different types of shampoos that are available and get some straight talk about the most popular hair care brand.

# THE SHAMPOO SECRET BEAUTY COMPANIES DON'T WANT YOU TO KNOW

*Corinne asks: I have a very sensitive scalp with fine hair and suffer from hair loss and dandruff. Dermatologists have advised me to use a clear gel shampoo that is clarifying or deep cleansing. So I've tried Suave Daily Clarifying Shampoo, Suave for Men Deep Cleaning Shampoo, Neutrogena Anti-residue Shampoo and Prell Classic Shampoo (original formula). I'm not happy with those choices and would like you to set me straight. What shampoo is going to work for me?*

While we hate to disagree with dermatologists, we don't understand why they recommended a deep-cleansing shampoo when you have dandruff. Deep-cleansing-type shampoos will remove the surface flakes, but only a dandruff shampoo can address the cause of flaking and itching. So we'd recommend finding a good dandruff shampoo instead of chasing deep-cleansing, clarifying and antiresidue products. This may seem confusing to you because the beauty companies tell you there are so many different kinds of shampoo. But in reality, every shampoo on the market falls into one of a few basic categories.

## THERE ARE ONLY FOUR MAIN SHAMPOO TYPES IN THE WORLD

All shampoo can be categorized by their basic function. So why are there what seem like thousands of products on the market, you ask? Because companies that sell shampoo need new ways to talk about their products to keep them sounding new and exciting. There's nothing wrong with companies being creative about their names and claims as long as they are honestly depicting what their products can do. But you can be a smarter consumer if you can see beyond the marketing hype and understand the functionality of these four basic shampoo types.

**1** **Deep cleansing shampoos** (*aka volumizing, clarifying, balancing, oil control and thickening*). These shampoos are designed to get gunk off your hair and scalp. They typically contain slightly higher levels of detergents so they foam and clean better. They include the examples above as well as salon products like Paul Mitchell Shampoo and Frederic Fekkai's Full Volume Shampoo.

**2** **Conditioning shampoos** (*aka moisturizing, 2-in-1, smoothing, antifrizz, strengthening, color care, straightening and hydrating*). These kinds of formulas are all about leaving a moisturizing agent, like silicone or polyquaternium-10, on the hair to smooth it. They are very good for dry hair, especially if you color-treat or heat-style, but they can weigh down fine hair. Good examples of this type include most of the Pantene formulas and some products from the L'Oreal Vive collection and Dove Advanced Care.

**3** **Baby shampoos** (aka *kids shampoo and tear-free*). These are milder, lower-foaming surfactant formulas that are designed not to sting or burn your eyes. They're better for babies but they don't clean hair as well. Johnson's Baby Shampoo is the classic example, but this category also includes Touch of an Angel and The Little Bath.

**4** **Antidandruff shampoos** (aka *anti-itch, flake control and dry scalp*). These are medicated shampoos that contain a drug ingredient that controls itching and flaking. In the United States these are considered to be over-the-counter (OTC) drugs. Head & Shoulders is the leading dandruff product; other examples include Nizoral Dandruff Shampoo and Redken Dandruff Control Shampoo.

## THE BOTTOM LINE

We hope this helps you better understand the marketing hype surrounding shampoo names. We're not saying that all shampoos are the same, or even that all shampoos in a given category type are the same. There are real performance differences so it's important for you to shop around and find a product that performs the way you like at a price that you can afford. Just don't get too hung up on the names the companies use to describe their products. That's the marketing part of the industry, not the science part.

# ARE SALON PRODUCTS IN REGULAR STORES THE SAME AS THOSE IN SALONS?

**Winnie wonders:** *Are the salon products that you buy at the local grocery store the same as the ones you can buy at a salon? I saw a news story that said products in stores are fakes.*

Salon products are no different than those sold in stores. Selling salon brands in places that aren't salons is called diversion. The truth is that these salon brands depend on "diverted" product to boost their sales. They want to have it both ways. They want to tell you that Paul Mitchell is a salon-only brand, which makes it seem more exclusive, but they also want the high-volume sales that they can get only through mass market outlets like your local Target or Walmart. Additionally, they don't want to anger their salon distributors because people are able to get the same stuff—but cheaper—in nonsalon outlets.

They make up this story of products being inferior. In nearly all cases, they are not. Here's how diversion works. Paul Mitchell hires a company to manufacture its products. Then Paul Mitchell salespeople get and fill orders from distributors. Distributors are legitimate businesses that sell directly to independent salons. The distributors can order as much as they want. They then sell it to the salons, which can then sell it to you.

## FOLLOW THE MONEY

Some of these distributors work directly with stores like CVS and Walgreens. So when these stores put in an order (a really big order, compared to a salon), the distributors just order more product from Paul Mitchell to fill the CVS order.

It's not likely that Paul Mitchell even questions the big orders because company salespeople like the extra sales. They turn a blind eye to what's going on just so they can express public "outrage" that their product is being sold at the local drugstore. This is a bunch of bunk.

The stuff you get at your local drugstore is every bit as good as the stuff you get at the salon. Don't be fooled. If the folks at Paul Mitchell really wanted to stop these sales, they would simply question their distributors and find out who is selling to these outlets.

The problem of counterfeiting is a real one, but it's not something that you'll find at large stores like Target. Target is not going to sell something contaminated because the company would be sued in a heartbeat. The places that are sketchy are the small shops (some salons) with the dust on top of the bottles. Those are the places you have to worry about.

## THE BOTTOM LINE

If you're buying a salon brand from a regular store, you can trust that there is no difference between that and the stuff you can get at a salon.

# ARE PAUL MITCHELL PRODUCTS MAKING YOUR HAIR BREAK?

**Joan asks:** *About a year ago my stylist started using Paul Mitchell products on me and I haven't loved my hair since! Now it's damaged and it breaks easily. My stylist blames me for using a flat iron. I know that doesn't help but I've used a flat iron for years and have never had this happen. She tells me that's because I had my hair colored so much. I have never had these problems until she switched to Paul Mitchell. Is it possible that his products made my hair start to break off and thin out?*

We see how you could think that Paul Mitchell made your hair go bad, but we doubt that's really what happened. Paul Mitchell products are not different enough from other products you've been using (except for probably costing more), so there is likely a different reason you're experiencing hair breakage. It is natural to leap to conclusions like this, but they are often incorrect.

Instead of worrying about Paul Mitchell, we'd blame three other factors for your hair problem:

**1** **Flat iron usage is very bad for your hair.** That's probably the most immediate cause of daily breakage. If you want less damage, consider ironing less frequently.

**2** **In the long run, the worst thing you can do is chemically color your hair.** Coloring breaks down the hair's protein, making it weaker. Frequent chemical processing literally pushes your hair to its "breaking point."

**3** **The first two factors are worsened because you're getting older and your hair is weaker.** As we age, our hair gets less dense and more prone to breakage. That's probably why you're seeing so much hair breakage recently—Father Time is catching up with you!

## WHAT TO DO

So, what can you do? Well, the shampoo doesn't matter much as long as you're using a conditioner. The Paul Mitchell conditioner is good, but so are many other cheaper, mass market brands like Fructis, Pantene and TRESemmé. You might consider using one of these every time you wash your hair. The conditioner should provide enough lubrication to the hair so that pulling on it with a comb does not break it. It may even provide some protection against the heat of the flat iron. If you're not using a conditioner, be sure to use a conditioning shampoo like Pantene 2-in-1. This should help slow your hair-breaking problem.

## THE BOTTOM LINE

In truth, heat, coloring and age are all conspiring against you to break your hair. You can't do anything about the aging process but if you stopped coloring and reduced the heat exposure, your hair would break less. Of course, then you might not like how it looks. Such is the price we pay for beauty!

# DOES OJON RESTORATIVE TREATMENT LIVE UP TO ITS HYPE?

**Alison asks:** *I am wondering what you think of the Ojon products, specifically their restorative hair treatment that claims a 52 percent improvement in the condition of very dry hair after just one use. Is this really any better than other products, and how does it work?*

Ojon's oil treatment consists of palm oil, fragrance and a few extracts. It's particularly interesting because recent research has shown that only *some* oils will actually penetrate the hair. Mineral oil and sunflower oil, for example, will not penetrate. But coconut oil (which is essentially the same as palm oil) will filter deep into the cortex because it is so similar to hair's natural lipids.

### OIL CONDITIONS HAIR

Why is that a big deal? Because the natural oils in your hair help make it flexible and waterproof. Washing your hair removes some of these natural oils. So it is possible that applying coconut oil to your hair can fight some of the effects of this oil loss. Once inside the hair, the oil serves as a re-fatting agent. However, this type of conditioning won't have much effect on the cuticle—the outer layer of hair—so you'll still need to use a good conditioner to smooth the hair and make it easier to comb.

Is that a good value? Well, that's another question. Any other coconut oil-based product should do about the same job and should be much cheaper. We don't recommend any specific brands, but look for products that feature coconut oil as the first ingredient.

Is there anything to Ojon's rain-forest hype? Well, its rain-forest story seems well-intentioned, but this ingredient isn't proven to work any better or any differently than non-rain-forest ingredients. Coconut trees only grow in tropical climates, but there's nothing special about trees from the rain forest. So if you like Ojon's products and you want to support their cause *and* you can afford the $55 for this product, then by all means buy it. But don't buy the product just because the company tells you its rain-forest extract is better.

## THE BOTTOM LINE

Based on recent scientific research, the palm oil used by Ojon should penetrate the hair. Therefore, it could protect your hair from overwashing. However, at $55, it's a bit pricey, so shop around for other coconut oil products because you may be able to get the same effect for less money.

# TWO NATURAL OILS THAT MAKE YOUR HAIR SHINY AND STRONG

*Shannon says:* I have been using coconut oil for a while and I feel my hair is stronger than it used to be. I'd like to keep using it and I want to add olive oil to make my hair shiny, but I'm worried that mixing the two oils will stop the coconut oil from penetrating. Is it OK to mix two oils on my hair?

Yes, studies have shown that coconut oil actually penetrates the hair to help make it stronger. And as it turns out, olive oil also has penetrating properties. Scientists at the Textile Research Institute tested olive oil, avocado oil, meadowfoam seed oil, sunflower oil and jojoba oil. Their results showed that straight-chain glycerides like olive oil easily penetrate into the hair. Polyunsaturated oils, like jojoba oil, are more open in their structure so they don't pass through the layers of cuticles very well.

What does that mean in plain English? Olive and avocado oils penetrate all the way into the hair shaft. Meadowfoam seed oil partially penetrates, and jojoba and sunflower oils don't penetrate at all. They're very superficial and don't really provide any practical benefit.

## THE BOTTOM LINE

Mixing coconut and olive oils shouldn't be a problem. In fact, it's possible that the olive/coconut oil combination might even penetrate hair better. We won't bore you with the details, but it has to do with mixed micelles. We'd start with a 50/50 mixture and see how that works for your hair.

# IS PANTENE GOOD OR BAD FOR YOUR HAIR?

*Kara says:* I've heard a lot of things about Pantene Pro-V's shampoo and conditioner. Many hairstylists swear on their hair dryers that it is awful for your hair. Supposedly, it coats your hair with plastic or wax to make it seem smooth, soft and shiny, instead of really moisturizing your hair. It also reportedly makes your scalp itchy and your hair fall out.

However, I've been using the Pantene Restoratives shampoo and conditioner for a few months now, and I find my hair less frizzy, more manageable, smoother and softer. I also use John Frieda Frizz-Ease and Pantene Pro-V Restoratives Frizz Control Ultra Smoothing Balm. So set me straight: Is Pantene good or bad for my hair?

Don't fall into the trap of believing everything your stylist tells you. While most stylists are very talented at cutting and styling hair, they're not very talented at interpreting cosmetic formulations.

The truth is that Pantene's shampoo and conditioner formulas are considered among the best in the industry by those of us in the cosmetic science side of the business. It makes sense if you think about it. Proctor & Gamble, makers of Pantene, have a *huge* research budget; certainly larger than any salon company. That means they can afford to dedicate resources to developing and testing the best formulas possible. We've seen Pantene formulas beat the pants off salon products in blind consumer testing. (The products are hidden, or blinded—not the consumers.)

## WHY IS PANTENE VILIFIED?

So why do stylists say that Pantene coats the hair with plastic, or makes it fall out? Because that's what they're told by the sales representatives for the salon companies. But it's just not true! Compare the ingredients lists for Pantene conditioner and any salon brand you can find. Even though the names vary, you'll see three basic types of ingredients:

Fatty alcohols (like cetyl and stearyl alcohol)

Conditioning ingredients (like stearamidopropylamine and quaternium-18)

Silicones (like dimethicone and cyclomethicone)

There's nary a plastic to be found in Pantene. And no, it doesn't make your hair fall out, either.

## THE BOTTOM LINE

You can choose whatever product you like—a retail brand like Pantene or a salon brand like Matrix. But shop around and make your own decisions based on your own experience. Don't pass on Pantene because of what a stylist tells you.

# DO CURLING SHAMPOOS REALLY WORK?

**Carol comments:** *I'd love to believe that those curling shampoos will really shape my thick hair. Will they?*

This is an easy one. Curling shampoos do *not* make your hair curly. In fact, if you read the labels carefully, some of them don't even *say* they'll make your hair curly!

## CHECK OUT THE BOTTLE

Let's take a look, shall we? Even the most blatant offender of the truth, Wash 'n Curl Shampoo, only *implies* that it will make your hair curly just by shampooing. Read the label carefully: It says it provides "the most beautiful curls with body, bounce and resilience after styling." Well, duh! If the shampoo only makes your hair curly *after* you style it, it's not really doing much for you, is it?

What else does Wash 'n Curl say? "Your hair will be extremely curl responsive… Even dry, damaged, color-treated hair will have the staying power of thick curly hair… Its special Curl Enhancers infuse hair with the Holding Power of naturally curly hair."

The only worthwhile part of this claim is that the shampoo does contain something that could be called a "curl enhancer." Looking at the ingredients list, we see that it does contain a polymer (acrylates/C10-30 alkyl acrylate crosspolymer), that *could* provide some styling benefits. But that would only work if it wasn't rinsed out!

Remember, just because a product contains an ingredient that does something doesn't mean that it does something in that product!

The rest of the claims are pretty much made up, as far as we can tell. There is not yet a shampoo technology that will measurably improve the holding power of your hair.

## OTHER CURLING SHAMPOOS

What about other products, you ask? Well, here are two more:

Neither KMS Curl Up Shampoo nor Marc Anthony Strictly Curls makes strong curling claims. KMS only promises to be your "curl's best friend," "start your style in the shower" and "boost boisterous curls while adding moisture and shine."

Marc, on the other hand, offers to protect color; repair dry, frizzy areas; and repel humidity to define shiny, soft curls. (*Define* curls is not really a very emphatic claim.) Aside from a little polyquaternium (a conditioning ingredient), neither of these products has any curling technology, either.

We could go on and on, but you get the picture. These shampoos don't have anything in them to make your hair curly. They don't even really do anything to prepare your hair for styling, other than getting it clean.

## THE BOTTOM LINE

If you really want curly hair, go buy some mousse or, God forbid, get a perm! Curling shampoos don't work.

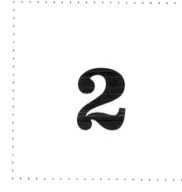

# 2

# TIPS ON CARING FOR YOUR HAIR

We all care about hair care products, but have you ever wondered what really works? In this chapter we'll give you tips on preventing split ends, drying hair properly, keeping it shiny, and we'll even explore how to keep your hair from smelling bad. If you want great-looking hair without spending a fortune, this chapter gives you the answers.

# DRYING DILEMMA: WHAT'S THE BEST WAY TO DRY YOUR HAIR?

*Angela asks:* I usually don't have the patience to blow-dry my hair completely, but my hairdresser said it's not good for my hair if I only half blow it dry and then let it finish drying by itself. Is it true?

We think this idea is kind of silly but we'll avoid the temptation to just tell you to get a new hairdresser and instead we'll try to present both sides of the story.

## TECHNICALLY SPEAKING

It's more damaging to blow-dry or towel-dry your hair than it is to let it air-dry. It's as simple as that. That's because heat from blow-dryers can mess with the natural lipid distribution in your hair *and* degrade the intercellular cement that holds the hair's protective cuticle in place. And the physical abrasion from towel-drying not only loosens healthy cuticles but can actually wear them away! So if you dry your hair a lot, you'll end up with less shine and more split ends.

## STYLISTICALLY SPEAKING

We assume a hairdresser would argue that blow-drying keeps your hair sleek and smooth and that air-drying makes it frizzy. At least this is what the hairdressers we have worked with think.

## THE BOTTOM LINE

It looks like the answer to your drying dilemma could come down to this: What's more important to you—avoiding damage or fighting frizz? Less damage is better for your long-term hair health, but nobody wants frizz. Only you can decide which to choose. But, hey, if you're *that* worried about frizz, you can always use a good smoothing product after you dry your hair. You can buy a few bottles of an effective frizz fighter, like John Frieda Frizz-Ease, for only twenty bucks!

# DOES ANTIDANDRUFF SHAMPOO REALLY WORK?

*Fran is feeling flaky:* What's your opinion of Burt's Bees Feelin' Flaky Shampoo? Checking out the ingredients list, it looks as if the formulation does a good job of avoiding skin irritants (except for the tea tree oil), but since it all gets washed off after a few seconds, I don't know how much good it could do. The ingredients are vegetable glycerin, lemon fruit water, sucrose cocoate, decyl polyglucose, willowbark extract, peppermint leaf extract (organic), willow leaf extract, burdock root extract, nettles leaf extract, yucca schidigera extract, cedar leaf oil, tea tree oil, lemon oil, rosemary oil, juniper oil, peppermint oil, xanthan gum (natural thickener), glucose, glucose oxidase and lactoperoxidase.

This is one of the shampoo issues that *really* make the Beauty Brains mad—false and misleading antidandruff claims. Some companies make it *appear* as though their products will control dandruff, but they really won't. The way companies do this may not be strictly illegal, but it certainly is unethical in our opinion. Let's look at this Burt's Bees product as an example. While we believe Burt's Bees generally produces high-quality products, the way they market their anti-dandruff shampoo is questionable.

## BURT'S BEES FEELIN' FLAKY SHAMPOO

According to drugstore.com, the full name of the product is Burt's Bees Doctor Burt's Herbal Treatment Shampoo with Cedar Leaf & Juniper Oil. Doctor Burt, huh? We know that the reference is tongue-in-cheek, but that sure sounds medicinal to us! Strike 1.

Below the name it describes the shampoo as *Feelin' Flaky?* with a question mark. In the context of cleaning hair and scalp, *flaky* is generally the term used to describe a symptom of dandruff. (Itchiness is another symptom.) Hmmm. Strike 2.

And finally the directions: "Wet hair, lather, rinse, then lather and rinse again. Shampoo at least three times a week for maximum effectiveness."

Maximum effectiveness? Again, sounds like they're promising some kind of sustained effect. If they're not talking about dandruff, what effectiveness are they talking about? Just getting your hair clean. That's lame—Strike 3!

While this product, and others like it, don't overtly claim to control dandruff, they seem to be making that implication.

## WHAT'S IN A REAL ANTIDANDRUFF SHAMPOO?

The truth is antidandruff shampoos contain active ingredients that treat the physiological causes of dandruff. How can you tell if a shampoo is really effective against dandruff? In the United States, look for active drug ingredients like zinc pyrithione (ZPT) or selenium sulfide. In Europe and a few other countries, look for octopyrox on the label. If you don't see some kind of legitimate active ingredient listed, it's not an effective antidandruff shampoo. Don't believe everything the cosmetics companies tell you!

## THE BOTTOM LINE

You ask "how much good" this product will do for you. Well, it will certainly get your hair clean. The primary surfactants (sucrose cocoate and decyl polyglucose) will see to that. And it won't dry your scalp out, either—those are pretty mild cleansers. But that's about it. It's not a medicated shampoo so it won't do anything to control dandruff.

# CAN YOU CLEAN YOUR HAIR WITH CONDITIONER?

*Nancy needs to know:* WEN *is a line of cleansing conditioners created by Hollywood hair stylist Chaz Dean. Dean believes that sulfates in most shampoos can be very damaging and stripping to hair, so he created these cleansing conditioners to clean hair without stripping it. Nancy wants to know if hair can really be better off in the long run by cleansing with a conditioner. And if it does work, would a regular drugstore conditioner produce the same effect?*

First of all, the idea of cleansing your hair with conditioner is not new and was not invented by Chaz. And no, he's not using any kind of revolutionary technology. Let's take a look at the ingredients:

> *water, glycerin, cetyl alcohol, rosemary leaf extract, wild cherry fruit extract, fig extract, chamomile extract, marigold flower extract, behentrimonium methosulfate, cetearyl alcohol, stearamidopropyl dimethylamine, amodimethicone, hydrolized wheat protein, polysorbate 60, panthenol, menthol, sweet almond oil, PEG-60 almond glycerides, methylisothiazolinone, methylchloroisothiazolinone, citric acid, essential oils.*

Looking at just the functional ingredients (leaving out extracts, preservatives and pH adjusters) leaves the following:

*glycerin, cetyl alcohol, behentrimonium methosulfate, cetearyl alcohol, stearamidopropyl dimethylamine (SADMA) and amodimethicone.*

## COMMON CONDITIONER

These are very common conditioning ingredients. Here's what they do: Glycerin can provide moisturization in a leave-on product, but it doesn't do anything for hair when it's rinsed out. Cetyl and cetearyl alcohol are thickening and emulsifying agents used to make a conditioner rich and creamy. Because they're oil-soluble they could, in theory, help lift some of the sebum off your hair and scalp. Behentrimonium methosulfate, SADMA and amodimethicone are very effective conditioning ingredients because they deposit on the hair.

## DOES IT WORK?

Could you clean your hair with this product? Sure, if your hair isn't very dirty, this could work pretty well. But so could any basic conditioner. In fact, we'd look for a conditioner that doesn't have any silicone in it, just to make sure it leaves as little on your hair as possible.

But what if you have greasy hair, or if you use hairspray, mousse, gel or putty? Then cleansing conditioners are not a very good idea. They don't have enough cleansing power to remove gunk from the hair. Chances are that cleansing with conditioner will leave your hair feeling dirty and weighed down.

## THE BOTTOM LINE

If you're really worried about drying your hair out by overshampooing, there's nothing wrong with skipping your shampoo and just rinsing with conditioner once in a while. But you don't need to spend $28 on a special product. A nice inexpensive drugstore brand like Suave or VO5 will do the same thing.

# WANT SHINY HAIR? AVOID THE DULLING DOZEN!

Naturally shiny hair has a cuticle that's smooth and flat; it's plumped up with water (about 10 to 15% by weight) and it's rich in natural oils that keep the whole thing "glued" together. Unfortunately, you're stealing shine from your hair every day and you probably don't even realize it. If you want good gloss, you should avoid these twelve things that can rob hair of shine. Or as we like to call them, the Dulling Dozen:

**1** **Flood damage**
Even "harmless" water can be a shine stealer. That's because too much moisture swells the hair shaft and causes the cuticle to buckle. The more frequently you wet your hair, the less shine you're likely to have.

**2** **Shampoo scrubbing**
Scrubbing bubbles seem cute but that rub-a-dub-dub lifts the cuticle even more. Using a conditioning shampoo can help because the hair shafts won't snag against each other when you're lathering up.

**3** **Careless underconditioning**
OK, we don't all need to condition *every* time we wash our hair. *But* if your hair is dry to begin with, it's much more likely to be damaged during and after styling if you skip conditioner. You're just giving shine away!

**4** **Death by towel-drying**
So now your hair is wet. What do you do? Blot, don't rub! A rough towel can cause an amazing amount of damage on wet hair.

**5** **The brush-off**
Don't fall for that old myth that you should brush your hair 100 strokes every night. While brushing does temporarily help by distributing natural oils, in the long run it strips off layers of cuticle and weakens hair.

**Hot-styling appliances**

Heat is the natural enemy of shine. That's because high temperatures damage the natural lipids (fancy word for oils) that help keep hair flexible and shiny. If you do decide to heat-style, use protection, like the silicone-containing TRESemmé Thermal Creations Heat Tamer spray.

 **Protective product residue**

Yes, you do need to use heat protection, but be careful what you wish for. Some leave-in creams and gels leave behind a dulling residue.

 **Color my world**

Chemical coloring is very damaging because it breaks down the inner structure of hair protein. Even if you use the special conditioner that comes with the coloring kit, your hair never fully recovers.

 **Wave bye-bye**

Permanent waving is another chemical process that's highly damaging.

 **Twist and shout**

Twisting and playing with your hair is a dangerous habit as far as shine is concerned. That's because the torsional forces (fancy word for twisting and bending) loosen the cuticles.

 **I dig a pony**

Wearing your hair in a ponytail may seem like a hassle-free style, but if you pull it back too tightly you may be creating microfractures in the hair that will reflect light unevenly and cause loss of shine.

 **Here somes the sun**

And with the sun comes damaging UV radiation that can wreak havoc on natural hair lipids like 18-methyl eicosanoic acid. Without these lipids, hair dulls quickly. If you can't stay out of the sun, make sure you're protecting your hair with a good conditioner.

# ARE HAIR EXTENSIONS KILLING YOUR HAIR?

**Wanda writes:** *I got hair extensions almost two years ago. I paid $4,000 for the kind that are put on individually with clips, which need to be put in and taken out with a tool that only salons have and they have to be adjusted every month.*

*After about nine months, as the stylist was adjusting the clips, I noticed that my hair was coming out along with the extensions! There was no more hair below the clip of hair extension hair. My hair was just gone. It all broke off at hundreds of different places where the clips were attached. It looked like a horror film!*

*I cried for months. Now my hair is still growing from my roots, but it's not getting longer. Is there anything I can do to help strengthen my hair and stop it from breaking? If I were a multimillionaire, would there be some way? Do movie stars have some way that we don't know about to repair their hair?*

Based on her description, Wanda probably has a condition known as traction alopecia, a type of hair loss that is caused by pulling on hair. In some cases this can be caused by wearing your hair in a ponytail; in this case it's caused by the weight of the extensions. Over a long period, this pulling stress can cause the follicle to atrophy and stop producing normal hairs. Depending on the intensity and duration of the stress, the follicle may or may not recover.

## FOLLICLE RECOVERY

If the extensions are removed in time, the follicles will recover and begin producing thick, strong hairs again. But if the follicles were permanently damaged, there's not much that can be done. Sadly, there is no secret millionaire's product that can solve the problem; there is no known medical treatment for late-stage traction alopecia.

One thing that *might* help increase hair strength, though, is treatment with pure coconut oil. Coconut oil is one of the few natural oils shown to penetrate the cortex and provide some strengthening effect to hair. It won't make hair grow any thicker, but it might help protect thinner, weaker strands.

# STRAIGHT TALK ABOUT STRAIGHTENING IRONS

*Corinne asks:* I'm in the market for a high-end straightening iron, and I feel completely overwhelmed by all the product choices out there! The major differences I see for most irons are the types of plates used, which include tourmaline/ceramic mix, ceramic and metal. While I'm presuming it's the high heat (some heat up to 450ºF) that helps straighten the hair shaft, how do these different plates benefit the hair? Are these newer kinds of straighteners with the tourmaline and ceramic healthier for your hair? I'm looking for an iron that works well, but doesn't completely wreck and fry my hair shaft.

The number of choices for hair appliances is, indeed, paralyzing! But you don't have to pay too much attention to all the hype about the different types of ironing plates. While it's true that more expensive irons can be made from higher-quality materials, that really just means that the heating element is more rugged and the plates are built to take wear and tear. Cheaper flat irons may have inferior plates that can't handle the heat and may snag your hair.

But whether it is tourmaline or ceramic, there's nothing about the composition of the plate material that makes it intrinsically healthier for your hair. And don't believe any of that crap about ionic straighteners. That's pure marketing hype without a shred of scientific validation.

## THE BOTTOM LINE

When buying a straightening iron, you'll need to pay a bit more for high-quality construction, but you don't need to pay extra for bogus scientific claims. There is no proof that tourmaline irons are better.

# HOW TO KILL LICE AND NOT YOUR HAIR

*Susan scratches her head:* I'm having a lice problem. I just want to know what's the most effective way to kill lice and nits and not dry or damage my hair in the process.

Head lice are tiny crawling insects about the size of a sesame seed or smaller. They have six clawed legs that they use to crawl over your hair; they cannot hop, jump or

# 9 TIPS TO STOP SMELLY HAIR

It seems that a lot of people are complaining about smelly hair, and the blogosphere is buzzing with tips on how to neutralize hair odors. Here are nine ways to get rid of the odor and keep your hair smelling great.

**1. Wash and condition your hair:** This may seem obvious, but it's the most thorough way to get your hair clean and odor-free.

**2. Hair wipes:** Hair wipes are like baby wipes made especially for your locks. Ted Gibson has an excellent product that should help remove any odor from your hair.

**3. Hair fragrance:** One way to get rid of an odor is to cover it up with some other odor. Hair fragrances are great for this purpose.

**4. Use your perfume:** If you can't find a "real" hair fragrance, just improvise with your favorite perfume or cologne. Just be sure not to use too much!

**5. Powder shampoo:** Instead of getting your hair wet, you can use a dry powder shampoo to add a little fragrance and remove the odor. Just sprinkle it in and brush the odors out.

**6. Leave-in conditioner or combing cream:** A touch of leave-in conditioner or another styling product can mask icky odors.

**7. Do a speedy, secret sink wash:** Wet your hands, take a *tiny* dab of liquid soap and run your fingers through your hair. Caution: This doesn't work on all hairstyles.

**8. Dryer sheets:** You'll cover up the odor *and* you'll get rid of embarrassing static cling.

**9. Use an antimicrobial shampoo:** This can help if your smelly scalp is caused by scalp fungus or bacteria.

fly. Lice lay eggs, also known as nits, which they glue to individual hair shafts. Lice live only on humans, not pets, and (here's the best part) they *feed on human blood!*

## NIT PICKING

The good news is that there several over-the-counter drug products that are effective against lice and nits. The bad news is that these products contain isopropyl alcohol, which can dry your hair. There are "natural" lice cures, but there is little or no data to prove that these are effective. The safest and surest way to get rid of lice and not damage your hair is to use a lice comb to pick the nits out one by one, but this is a very tedious and time-consuming process.

Recently, there was a study done by researchers at the University of Utah in which they created a steam-cleaning device (a cross between a vacuum cleaner and a hair dryer) to kill lice. It's not even available to the public yet, but it could prove to be an interesting new treatment.

## BEST LICE TREATMENT

Which treatment method is best? Rather than spelling out all the pros and cons of each method here, go to HeadLice.org for a thorough question-and-answer page. And if you do decide to use the lice-killing shampoo, make sure you follow that with a good conditioner to counteract the drying effects of the alcohol.

# 3 HAIR MYTHS

While your mom, friends and stylist are well-meaning when they give you advice about hair products, they may not be giving you accurate, science-based information. We do that here as we explore some common myths about hair products and let you know whether they are true or not. Should you really avoid silicone? Do certain products leave plastic on your hair? Read on to find out.

# ARE YOU SPENDING TOO MUCH ON CONDITIONER?

**Christine queries:** *Will a more expensive conditioner make my hair stronger? I'm a science teacher, so don't spare me the technical details!*

Expensive does *not* always mean better when it comes to hair and skin care products, but to explain further, we'll have to fill you in on how conditioners work.

## HOW DO CONDITIONERS STRENGTHEN HAIR?

The outer layer of the hair consists of overlapping scales, called cuticles. These cuticles are like the shingles on the roof of your house—they protect what's beneath it. As your hair is damaged from washing and drying and combing and brushing and perming and coloring, the cuticle starts to wear away. When this happens, your hair is broken more easily.

Conditioners strengthen hair in two ways. The most important thing they do is smooth the cuticle and help keep it in place. The "strengthening" effect can be shown by measuring combing force. The other effect is internal. Some ingredients, like panthenol, penetrate into the cortex, the middle part of the hair. By interacting with the proteins in the cortex, these conditioners can improve the tensile strength of hair. This type of strength is measured with an instrument that pulls on individual hair fibers (after they've been removed from your head, of course!) and measures how much force it takes for the hair to break.

## ARE EXPENSIVE CONDITIONERS BETTER?

So do expensive conditioners strengthen hair better than cheap ones? Not necessarily. The very, very cheap conditioners typically rely on one or two conditioning agents to do the job. And they usually can't afford to use silicones, which are among the most effective smoothing agents. So, chances are, if you're only spending a buck or two on your conditioner, you're not getting the best product.

But once you get up in price to the $4 or $5 conditioners, the differences in strengthening are less significant. For example, Pantene and TRESemmé are among the best conditioners we've ever tested and they're certainly not that expensive. Most mid- or high-priced conditioners will do a pretty good job of lubricating your hair to prevent breakage.

## CAN A CONDITIONER BE *TOO* EXPENSIVE?

What about the conditioners that are $30 per bottle? They use the same basic types of ingredients as products that cost $10 or less. They may cost three times more, but they certainly don't strengthen your hair three times more! But, as we always say, you should buy what you like and what you can afford. If you really like the way Frederic Fekkai's Overnight Hair Repair makes your hair feel, and you can afford the $195 per bottle, then go for it. (Yes, that's right—it's nearly $200!) But don't buy it just because you think that it will make your hair stronger than a less expensive brand. It won't.

## THE BOTTOM LINE

Picking the right conditioner is a personal thing. There are literally thousands of combinations of ingredients out there and it's tough to know which one is best for you. So talk to your friends who have similar hair types. Or just experiment until you find something that feels good. But *don't* be tricked into spending more money than you want to.

# ARE SILICONES BAD FOR YOUR HAIR?

**Bonnie is confused:** *There seems to be a lot of conflicting information about silicone-heavy hair products, and whether or not they help make hair soft and silky. I'm concerned about buildup and having my hair dry out. Also, how do more natural alternatives, like coconut and sweet almond oil, compare?*

In general, silicones work by covering hair with a thin, hydrophobic (waterproof) coating. This coating serves several purposes: It helps reduce the porosity of the hair, which makes it less likely to absorb humidity; it helps reduce moisture loss from the inside of the hair; and it lubricates the surface of the hair so it feels smoother and can be combed more easily.

## PROPERTIES OF SILICONES

The properties vary depending on which silicone is in the formula. Some silicones leave a heavy coating on the hair that can be hard to wash off. Others are very water-soluble and don't build up at all. Dimethicone (sometimes called simethicone), for example, is the heaviest of all silicones used for hair care. It provides the most smoothing effect, but it is also the hardest to wash out. Cyclomethicone, on the other hand, gives a great slippery feeling while you're rinsing your hair, but it evaporates quickly, leaving nothing behind.

Some natural oils are effective conditioners. Coconut oil, for example, doesn't provide the same surface smoothing as silicones, but it has been shown to penetrate hair and plasticize the cortex, making hair stronger. (This isn't true of all natural oils, however.) So oils are useful ingredients, but they're not direct replacements for silicones.

## THE BOTTOM LINE

It's tough to tell which silicones are the best simply from reading the label because there are so many types of silicones and they can be used in combination with each other. You can't simply say that all silicones are bad. Some women will find silicones too heavy for their hair; others will love the soft, conditioned feel they provide. You have to experiment to find what's right for you.

# WHAT'S THE DIFFERENCE BETWEEN A SILICONE AND A POLYQUAT?

*Jackie just needs to know:* What's the difference between a silicone and a polyquat? Do both coat and stay on the hair? Do they both need to be removed by sulfates? Do they both tend to build up on the hair?

Silicones and polyquats are ingredients found in both shampoos and conditioners. They are put in formulas to offset the drying effects of detergents, improving hair by making it easier to comb, making it feel softer, increasing shine and reducing static flyaway. They really are amazing materials. The primary difference between them is their chemical composition and the way they stay on the hair.

**\*\*Caution: Science talk coming up…**

### SILICONES ARE MADE OF SILICON

Silicones (or "cones") are molecules that have silicon in them. The silicone, which is typically derived from sand, reacts with oxygen, carbon and hydrogen to make useful materials. Ingredients like dimethicone and cyclomethicone are naturally slippery and shiny, which is why they are excellent for hair.

## POLYQUATS ARE MADE OF HYDROCARBONS

Polyquats are molecules that are composed primarily of carbon, hydrogen and nitrogen. The *quat* part refers to the fact that they contain a positively charged nitrogen atom and the *poly* part refers to the fact that they are polymers. They also have a slippery effect and can smooth hair while reducing static charge.

## BOTH STAY ON HAIR, BUT IN DIFFERENT WAYS

Because of the different chemistry of polyquats and silicones, each of these compounds uses a different method to stay on the hair. On hair, the damaged portions are typically negatively charged. The positive charges on the polyquat allow it to stick to these negative sites on the hair. It is a bit like two magnets being attracted to each other.

Silicones are not usually charged, but stay on the hair because of their incompatibility with water. If you put a drop of silicone in water, it will not dissolve, no matter how much you stir it. When a silicone product is put on your hair, it deposits and resists being washed off.

## DETERGENTS ARE NEEDED TO REMOVE THEM

Since silicones and polyquats stick to hair, they need more than just water to remove them. In fact, silicones can stick to hair so well that they may require multiple shampooings before they are removed. Similarly, some polyquats may be difficult to remove from hair. While a sulfate shampoo isn't required to remove them, sulfates are your best bet.

## BOTH MAY BUILD UP ON HAIR

Depending on the type of molecule, both silicones and polyquats may build up on your hair. Dimethicone is one of the most difficult silicones to remove and multiple use of products with it can make your hair look dull and weighed down over time. Cyclomethicone, on the other hand, evaporates from hair like water and will not cause the same problems. Polyquats do not build up as much, but still require occasional washing with a polyquat-free shampoo.

## THE BOTTOM LINE

Silicones and polyquats are different materials but they both stay on hair and can build up over time. It is a good idea to wash your hair once a week with a shampoo that doesn't contain either one in order to prevent buildup and keep your hair looking fresh, shiny and manageable.

# WHY DOES SILICONE BUILD UP ON HAIR?

When it comes to buildup, the type of silicone (and how much is used) is more important than if it's used in a leave-on styler or a rinse-off conditioner. There are *many* types of silicone with scientific names that can be confusing, so let's look at a few common examples.

## NO BUILDUP

One of the most common types of silicone is called "cyclic" because the chain of silicone atoms that composes this kind is linked together in a ring structure. This type of silicone evaporates and won't build up on your hair at all. It gives a silky-smooth feel and leaves the hair with incredible slip when wet. It's used in both leave-on stylers and rinse-off conditioners and is commonly called cyclomethicone or cyclopentasiloxane.

## VERY LITTLE BUILDUP

Another type of silicone is designed to be water-soluble. This kind provides very light conditioning and is unlikely to build up because it washes away easily with water. It is often used in conditioning shampoos. Look for *polyol* in the name, as in dimethicone copolyol.

## MODERATE TO HEAVY BUILDUP

There is a different kind of silicone that is chemically modified to stick to your hair better. That means it conditions well, but it can also be more challenging to remove. This kind generally has *amo*, *amine* or *amino* somewhere in the name. For example, amodimethicone is commonly used in leave-in conditioners.

## POTENTIALLY HEAVY BUILDUP

Finally, perhaps the most powerful type of silicone is referred to as a silicone oil. It comes in many different forms but is typically used at very high molecular weights to make it highly waterproof, so it provides good shine to the hair. Because it's so water-insoluble, it can be very tough to wash off, depending, of course, on how much you have on your hair. Typically, this is used in rinse-off products. Look for it on the ingredients list as dimethicone.

# IS BABY SHAMPOO GOOD FOR ADULT HAIR?

*Sylvia asks:* Are baby shampoos sufficient to clean adult hair? I know they are sulfate-free and I have been looking for this type of shampoo to minimize the drying effect from shampoos with sulfates.

There is a lot of misinformation out there about sodium lauryl sulfate (SLS) and shampoo.

## IS SLS BAD?

First of all, don't believe all the urban legends about SLS causing cancer or being bad for you because it's used in garage cleaners. We've debunked this myth in chapter 10. Most people can use sodium lauryl sulfate or ammonium lauryl sulfate shampoos without any problem whatsoever.

*But,* some people do find that SLS can dry out their scalp. Those people should consider SLS's milder cousin SLES (short for sodium lauryl ether sulfate) or they should consider using sulfate-free shampoos.

## ARE BABY SHAMPOOS GOOD CLEANSERS?

Baby shampoos are good examples of sulfate-free formulas. Instead of SLS, they contain materials known as amphoteric surfactants, which are less drying to skin and milder to the eye. (Hence the "no more tears" claim of many baby shampoos.)

The downside to these types of formulations is that they don't clean as well as the stronger detergent systems. While SLS is a *very* good cleansing agent that can remove sweat, dirt, styling product residue and scalp oils, baby shampoo formulas are not so effective.

## WHY NOT BABY YOURSELF?

Is this a problem? It depends. If you're using a ton of styling products, you might have to shampoo your hair multiple times with baby shampoo to get it as clean as with an SLS-based product. That's not such a bad trade-off if your scalp is really dried out.

## THE BOTTOM LINE

Sulfate-free baby shampoos can clean hair adequately enough for most adults. They are less drying and irritating but will not foam as well, so you might not think they are working. If you're curious, we recommend trying baby shampoo for a week or two to see if you like the effect. If not, you can always switch back.

# CAN YOU REALLY REBUILD YOUR HAIR?

*Amanda asks: What is the deal with "restructuring" treatments for hair? I get that the vague concept is to "restore proteins" to your hair or some gobbledygook, but isn't hair essentially dead? Can a restructuring treatment really force-feed amino acids or whatever into our manes?*

The Beauty Brains love Amanda's skepticism, because the idea of being able to slather on a hair restructuring treatment to actually re-form hair is ridiculous. True, hair is made of amino acids and putting them on hair may provide some minor benefit. But it won't restructure, restore or rebuild the hair. This would be a bit like trying to repair a weather-worn Kate Spade bag by pouring a basket of thread and fabric on it. Sure, the stylish sack is made of thread and fabric, but you can't just randomly put them on the worn bag and expect to get a new purse.

## RESTRUCTURE HAIR?

It's the same with hair and amino acids. To restructure the hair, the amino acids would have to be chemically arranged in a specific way. This arrangement can only be done in the hair follicle when the hair is growing. After that, nothing can be done except coat the hair with a good conditioner that mitigates some of the signs of damage. So what are these restructuring treatments? In essence, they are just glorified rinse-out conditioners.

Let's take a look at the ingredients in a "restructuring" conditioner: *purified water, glyceryl stearate, PEG-100 stearate, stearamidopropyl dimethylamine, cetyl alcohol, propylene glycol, stearyl alcohol, dimethicone, triamino copper nutritional complex, hydroxyethylcellulose, panthenol, aloe vera gel, soydimonium hydroxypropyl hydrolyzed wheat protein, hydrolyzed keratin, citric acid, methylparaben, fragrance, disodium EDTA, propylparaben, peppermint oil, tocopheryl acetate, cholecalciferol, retinyl palmitate, vegetable oil, FD&C Blue 1, D&C Red 33.*

The rules of cosmetic labeling require that ingredients be listed in order of concentration above 1 percent. In general, the more of an ingredient in the formula, the greater the impact it has on the product. The ingredients near the end of the list are just put in there to make a nice marketing story or are color, fragrance or preservatives.

In this formula, some of the main working ingredients are stearamidopropyl dimethylamine, cetyl alcohol, stearyl alcohol and dimethicone.

But then take a look at the ingredients list in a regular rinse-out conditioner: *water, stearyl alcohol, cyclopentasiloxane, cetyl alcohol, stearamidopropyl dimethylamine, glutamic acid, dimethicone, benzyl alcohol, fragrance, panthenyl ethyl ether, EDTA, panthenol, methylchloroisothiazolinone, methylisothiazolinone.*

Notice any similarities? The main working ingredients here are stearyl alcohol, cyclopentasiloxane, cetyl alcohol, stearamidopropyl dimethylamine and dimethicone.

## THE BOTTOM LINE

A restructuring conditioner will not rebuild your hair any better than a standard rinse-out formula. And it certainly won't rebuild your hair better than thread and fabric would rebuild a worn-out Kate Spade bag.

# DO YOU REALLY NEED TO PUT PROTEIN ON YOUR HAIR?

**Debbie says:** *I've been told that hair needs protein and moisturization to stay healthy. So for protein I use Mane 'n Tail and for moisturizing I use hair cholesterol products (like Le Kair, Queen Helene) and coconut oil. Is this good for my hair or could I be causing any kind of long-term damage?*

These conditioners won't damage hair. You might find that your hair is weighed down if you're using them all at once, but other than that they won't do anything bad to your hair. So if you like the way these conditioners make your hair feel, then keep using them any way you like. The real question here is does hair need both protein and moisturizer? The answer is yes and no.

## *YES,* HAIR NEEDS MOISTURE

That just means you need to keep your hair from drying out, which is the whole idea behind conditioners. You can moisturize by adding water (which doesn't really stay in your hair very long) or you can moisturize by fighting the effects of dryness. That's what any good conditioner does. Conditioners, like Le Kair and Queen Helene, work by smoothing the outer layers of your hair, the part called the cuticle. If you don't keep the cuticles "glued down," they tend to come loose and fall off. Whenever you're doing anything to your hair (including washing, drying, styling or coloring), you are causing some degree of damage to those cuticles. What a good conditioner does is smooth the cuticles, forming a protective layer over them so they don't become as damaged.

### NO, HAIR DOESN'T NEED PROTEIN

Although hair is made of protein, it's dead. So putting protein on top of the protein in your hair doesn't make it "healthy." But the right kind of proteins used at the right levels can act as conditioning agents that form a protective film on the hair. So it's not that your hair needs protein, it's that it needs *something* to form that protective layer.

Proteins will do it to some extent, but there are other ingredients, like fatty quaternium compounds or silicones, that will work even better. So protein conditioners like Mane 'n Tail are good for your hair, but not necessarily *because* they contain protein.

### THE BOTTOM LINE

There are many, many great hair conditioners on the market that will moisturize your hair. Mane 'n Tail, Le Kair and Queen Helene won't do anything bad to your hair. The important thing is to find the products that feel right for your hair and that you can afford. But don't worry too much about special ingredients like proteins. And by the way, coconut oil has an added benefit. It penetrates through the cuticle to strengthen the inside part of the hair called the cortex. See page 7 for more about this.

# HOW MUCH HAIR LOSS IS NORMAL?

*Janelle asks:* Every time I shampoo, I tend to lose around 40 strands and the same again when combing. Is this normal? And does the shampoo I use have anything to do with how much hair I lose?

One of the things we forget is that we are animals and, just like all other animals, we shed. So you shouldn't be surprised that you lose some hair every day. But is 40 to 100 strands normal?

On the average person's head (assuming there aren't any bald spots), there is an average of 100,000 hairs. Feel free to count them if you like…we'll wait. This is somewhat related to your natural hair color: Brunettes average about 120,000 hairs while redheads have only 90,000. The number of hairs is strictly controlled by your genetic makeup, which means there is nothing you can do to increase the number of hairs on your head.

At any given moment, each hair follicle on your head is in one of three growth phases. The anagen phase is when the hair is growing and actually getting longer. This can last anywhere from two to seven years. The catagen phase is a transitional phase, when growth slows and eventually stops. The telogen phase is the final phase, in which growth has completely stopped and the hair is vulnerable to falling out. The hairs that you naturally shed are all in the telogen phase.

Studies have shown that you should expect to shed approximately 0.1 percent of your hair each day. That means you lose 100 hairs every day. This is almost exactly the amount you are asking about. And remember: This is a biological rate; it has nothing to do with the shampoo you use.

The only effect hair products will have on the amount of hair you lose is that they may make you notice more lost hairs. Washing and styling involve lots of movement, so hairs will be more likely to fall out if they are ready. However, this will be true of any hair care brand.

## THE BOTTOM LINE

Hair falls out naturally and the brand of shampoo you use will not have any added effect.

# WHY DO GRAY HAIRS LOOK AND FEEL DIFFERENT?

*Tiffany wants to know:* Why do my gray hairs seem more kinky and unruly compared to the rest of my hair?

Gray hair looks gray because it has lost its melanin, which gives hair its color. Melanin is naturally produced in the hair follicle and "injected" into the hair fibers as the protein is formed and pushed out of the head. It's the same kind of melanin that gives your skin its color. Two basic types of melanin (eumelanin and pheomelanin) are responsible for every hair color from brown and black to blond and red.

No one knows why hair follicles stop producing melanin. Genetics mostly. There comes a point where the melanocytes (the melanin-producing cells) just stop producing. Thus you get gray hair.

# WILL HAIR DYE GIVE YOU CANCER?

Every so often you hear about how chemicals in your cosmetics are responsible for cancer, birth defects or even autism. Unfortunately, the sources for these conclusions are rarely cited and, when they are, they are typically a biased political committee or marketing group.

An article titled "Can dyeing your hair really give you cancer?" recently caught our eye. The article discussed a major conference that was being held in Belfast in which the long-term link between bladder cancer and people with dyed hair was being discussed. It stated:

> Evidence exists to indicate regular and long-term use of hair dyes can
> be associated with the development of the cancer, which kills more than
> 4,000 in the UK each year.

Now, if this article was all you read on the subject, you might conclude that hair dye causes bladder cancer. You might also get the impression that experts are in agreement. After all, they did get their information from Questor, a European environmental research center.

Being the skeptical Beauty Brains that we are, we went to see what the medical journals had to say on the subject. A search of "hair dye" resulted in 649 hits. The most current research is useful for answering questions like these; review articles are best. Review articles are designed to summarize all the work that has been published before.

An article about hair dye and cancer published in late 2006 in the *Journal of Toxicology and Environmental Health* concludes:

> *Results for bladder cancer studies suggest that subsets of the population may be genetically susceptible to hair dye exposures, but these findings are based on small subgroups in one well-designed case-control study. Replication of these findings is needed to determine whether the reported associations are real or spurious.*

This is a bit different than the definitive bladder cancer/hair dye link suggested in the newspaper article. Essentially, the researchers say certain genetically predisposed people may have issues, but even this isn't a certainty. A more thorough study is needed. But the important implication is that for most people, this isn't a problem. Hair dye will not cause cancer.

What you read, see or hear in the mainstream media rarely tells the whole story. When it comes to issues about health and safety you would not be wrong to immediately reject their conclusions. If you want to know the real story, do a little research for yourself using the least biased sources you can find. Research in this case would find that the majority of studies show no established link between hair dye and cancer. So feel free to color with abandon.

For a more thorough summary of the cancer/hair color research, read this article published in the *Journal of the American Medical Association:* http://jama.ama-assn.org/cgi/content/abstract/293/20/2516.

## CAN YOU SLOW IT DOWN?

No one has figured out how to do this yet. And the truth is that only the pharmaceutical companies would be looking for the solution anyway. Cosmetics companies focus on things that do not react with your body. I'm not sure if there will be a solution to this problem anytime soon. (By the way, there are products out there like Reminex that claim to restore melanin production, but we've seen no data to indicate that they work.)

## WHY DO PEOPLE THINK GRAY HAIR IS SO DIFFERENT?

There are probably two reasons: First, we know that as you age, the follicles produce less of their natural lubricating oils. That can make hair feel dry and coarse. Second, gray hairs are just easier to notice because of the color difference. Think about all the hairs on your head that are unruly. Those that are the same color as the rest of your hair simply don't get noticed.

## THE BOTTOM LINE

There is no solid data to show that gray hair has a different physical structure that makes it feel more kinky and unruly. In fact, we've seen experiments that show if people close their eyes they cannot feel a difference between gray hair and "normal" hair.

# WILL HONEY AND CINNAMON HELP STOP HAIR FROM FALLING OUT BUT TURN HAIR GRAY?

*Sosina says:* I read on the internet that applying honey and cinnamon to hair is good for treating hair loss. But people say that honey makes hair gray. Which one is true?

The internet is a wonderful tool, but remember anyone can write anything, and you never know what is really true. (Unless you're reading the Beauty Brains, that is.)

## WHAT DOES HONEY DO ON HAIR?

Honey is a humectant, which means it has a tendency to hold on to water molecules. This is a desirable property in a moisturizer, especially one designed for skin. But unlike skin, hair is not alive and it doesn't need as much moisture as skin does.

Honey is not a good lubricant, so it doesn't have any benefit for making hair slippery and smooth. In fact, it's the opposite of slippery—it's sticky because it's basically a sugary solution. (Rub some between your fingers and you'll see!) It will not smooth your cuticles or help a comb pass through your hair without damaging it. So any moisture-grabbing benefits that honey might give your hair are offset by its stickiness. The bottom line is that honey is not good for conditioning your hair.

But what about hair loss and graying?

## HONEY AND HAIR LOSS

Hair loss is one of the most vexing cosmetic problems facing both men and women. Hundreds of thousands of materials have been suggested as a treatment but the truth is the only topical treatment that has been proven to work is Minoxidil. And even this is not effective for the majority of people. There is no proof that honey prevents hair loss and there isn't even any scientific reason that it would work.

## HONEY AND GRAY HAIR

Gray hair is the result of melanocytes (pigment-producing cells) in your hair follicles shutting down. Literally, your gray hair has no pigment, thus no color. Fortunately, exposure to honey will not cause your hair to turn gray. In fact, it might even help stain your hair to make it darker.

## CINNAMON AND YOUR HAIR

While honey is primarily sugar, cinnamon is made up of a variety of bioactive materials, including cinnamaldehyde, essential oils and antioxidants. If either honey or cinnamon would have an effect on hair loss, cinnamon certainly would be a better candidate. There is some evidence that cinnamon has an anti-inflammatory effect. Another anti-inflammatory ingredient, silanediol salicylate, is currently being studied for its potential to reduce hair loss, raising the possibility that cinnamon might also help in a similar way. However, there is still no solid proof that anti-inflammatory agents help stop or reverse hair loss.

## THE BOTTOM LINE

Neither honey nor cinnamon has been proven to help stop hair loss or turn hair gray, but if you are going to try one, go for cinnamon. At least it has the potential to do something.

# ARE THE PICTURES ON THE BACK OF THE SHAMPOO BOTTLE ACCURATE?

*Rosanna requests:* On the back of many Pantene shampoo bottles, there are pictures—one that shows damaged hair and one that shows repaired hair after the use of Pantene. Are those pictures realistic and, if so, how long does it take for the repair to take place?

Pantene has been the market leader in shampoo for over ten years, partly because it is an inexpensive and excellently formulated product. However, to maintain this kind of market dominance, you need more than great technology. You need the best marketing in the industry and that's what Procter & Gamble (the makers of Pantene) has.

## PANTENE SMOOTHES HAIR FIBERS

Believe it or not, the pictures on the back of Pantene's bottles do give a reasonable representation of what is happening on your hair. What is shown are two pictures of hair strands—one strand has cuticles that are jagged and lifted up, the other strand is smooth and nicer-looking. The message you are supposed to get from this is that by using Pantene shampoo and conditioner, your hair will be softer, smoother and shinier. Is it true? It is true that the cuticles (the outer layer of a hair fiber) of damaged hair will look jagged and lift up from the fiber. The image is an artist's rendition of a close-up microscopic view of the hair. When a fiber is treated with a conditioning shampoo like Pantene, it leaves a coating of silicone and polyquat that "glues" down the cuticles and makes the hair look smooth.

This effect is immediate and doesn't require weeks of product use. But Pantene's advertising claims that your hair gets better after a month is more story than fact. Hair gets better right away. There could be a minor improvement over time but, for the most part, as soon as you apply Pantene you'll get the benefit.

We should mention that almost any conditioning shampoo could put a similar picture on the back of its shampoo bottles. Any shampoo that leaves a coating of silicone or polyquat will have this smoothing effect on the cuticles. Also, any conditioner will have this effect, too.

## THE BOTTOM LINE

The images on the back of a Pantene shampoo bottle do demonstrate how the product actually works. The effect is immediate and one you can get from almost any moisturizing or 2-in-1 shampoo.

# WHAT'S THE DIFFERENCE BETWEEN ALL THOSE HAIR COLOR PRODUCTS?

*Sandy wants to know:* *What do all those different hair color products do? Also, do they damage your hair if you add highlights?*

Highlights, lowlights, washable, semipermanent, demipermanent, permanent! With all the different hair color products out there, it's no wonder people are confused. Add to that all the different color shades and it's enough to make you give up.

## TYPES OF HAIR COLOR PRODUCTS

Hair colors are all classified by the length of time they will last in your hair. Here they are in order of shortest-lasting color to longest.

**1** **Washable:** These are temporary dyes and stains that wash off relatively easily with shampoo. They are also called "deposit only" colors. The benefit of this type of coloring is that it does not damage hair. The drawback is that the color does not look as good or last as long.

**2** **Semipermanent:** If you are unsure about a new hair color, the semipermanent route may be the way to go. These products deposit color on and just below the surface of hair. They do not break down your natural color so they can only be used to make your hair darker. Demipermanent hair colors use the same basic technology but last a little longer. They look good and do not damage your hair as much as permanent colors, but they also don't last as long.

**3** **Permanent:** These colors completely change the hair and can make even the darkest brunette into a bleach-blond bombshell. They work in a multiple-step chemical process. First, the color that is already in the hair is chemically broken down with hydrogen peroxide. This step also has the effect of opening up the hair "pores" so the color molecules can get in. Next, color is applied and allowed to chemically react. As it reacts, the color molecules get too big and become locked inside the hair shaft. This is how the color becomes permanent. This method gives you the most natural, longest-lasting hair color possible. Unfortunately, it is also the most damaging to hair. There's always a trade-off.

**4** **Highlights:** Blond highlights are the result of bleaching hair in a controlled way. Aluminum foil is often used to keep the peroxide bleach away from hairs that are not to be colored. The process is permanent (until your hair grows out, of course) and highly damaging. But it does make your hair look great!

## DOES HIGHLIGHTING HURT HAIR?

Permanent highlights chemically break down hair, so they definitely make it weaker. But most people like how highlights look, so they are willing to suffer a little damage. Washable highlights are based on temporary colors and do not damage hair. If you are unsure whether you will like having highlights, starting with the washable kind is an excellent idea. If you want the look to last longer than a couple of days, however, you'll have to get permanent highlights.

## THE BOTTOM LINE

While permanent hair color is damaging, it looks better and lasts longer than the semipermanent and washable options. If you want your hair color to look as good as it can, go for a permanent color and have it applied by a skilled hairdresser.

# IS A RELAXER THE ONLY WAY TO GET HAIR REALLY STRAIGHT?

*Valerie asks:* Is there anything out there in the market to straighten my hair without using a harsh chemical relaxer?

The quest for straight hair has led people to try everything from pulling, ironing and blow-drying to chemical treatments. Chemical relaxers have a number of drawbacks, including being inconvenient, expensive and, worse, painful. Relaxers are the most damaging cosmetic treatment you can do to hair.

Unfortunately, there is nothing on the market that works as well or lasts as long as chemical relaxers. However, there are at least five other things you can try to get straight hair that won't cause as much damage. These include the following:

**Hairdressings and silicone creams:** Products to control your hair shape have been around for over a hundred years. They contain oily materials like petrolatum, mineral oil and lanolin, which coat hair and prevent it from taking its natural shape. Silicone creams are also available and contain materials like dimethicone or cyclomethicone. The product is put on damp hair and combed straight. VO5 Hairdressing is the most famous of these types of products.

Performance These treatments work well for all types of hair, are nondamaging and are relatively inexpensive. On the other hand, they leave hair feeling greasy, looking unnatural and they only last until your next wash.

**Brushing, blow-drying and styling:** When hair gets wet, it straightens out. If you can hold the hair in that shape while drying it, you can keep it straight. To aid in this process, styling products like gels, mousses and pomades can all be used. These products will add an additional polymer coating on hair to keep it straight.

Performance This method can be effective but requires a lot of time and some skill in applying the product and shaping your hair. It is minimally damaging and can lead to a natural look. However, the effect doesn't work on all hair types and lasts only until your next wash. This is much easier if done by a stylist.

**Flat iron:** If you have really curly hair and the blow-drying + brushing method doesn't work, a flat iron might. Used on clean, dry hair, it gets hair straight in the same way as blow-drying, but it is more intense and effective on nearly all hair types, especially dry hair.

Performance Flat irons work with almost any hair type and can give a nice, natural look if you know what you are doing. However, they are damaging to hair and hair will frizz out when humidity is high if you don't use a styling product, too. The results are temporary and have to be redone any time your hair gets wet.

**Brazilian hair straightening:** This is a chemical treatment in which a stylist applies a keratin protein formula and uses a flat iron to get your hair straight. Theoretically, the protein crystallizes on your hair, which helps keep it straight for many weeks. To retain the look, you need to avoid washing your hair.

Performance Although this method works, at $150 and up per treatment, it hardly seems worth it. You can't wash your hair or it will return to its natural, curly state. There's also the issue of a significant amount of formaldehyde being released during the process. It is probably not a problem for occasional use, but imagine your poor stylist! You can get the same effect using a flat iron, styling products and less frequent hair washing, so it's probably not worth the money.

**Japanese straightening system:** This is a more permanent way to remove the curls from your hair. At $500 and up per treatment, it is the most expensive of all the methods listed. During the Japanese straightening system, the stylist applies a special formula consisting of reducing agents like Thioglycolates. Then a flat iron and a neutralizing solution make the hair straight. With proper care the effect can last for six months.

Performance The high price of this procedure has kept most people away from repeat procedures. It uses a process similar to traditional relaxers and is just as damaging. If you are looking for a replacement for relaxers, this is not a good choice.

**Relaxers:** No doubt about it—relaxers are the most effective and permanent way to take curls out of hair. They are more effective and less expensive than either the

Brazilian or the Japanese systems. Relaxers employ a chemical like sodium hydroxide to break down hair bonds and permanently change the structure.

Performance Relaxers are the most damaging hair treatment, so your hair will break more easily and feel dry. Also, your curly hair will grow back so you'll need to continue to relax your hair every six weeks to keep it straight.

## THE BOTTOM LINE

At the moment, there is no less-harsh treatment that works as well as a relaxer. Blow-dryers, styling products and flat irons can mimic the results, but they take a long time and are short-lasting.

# WHY DOES SHAMPOO HAVE MEAT TENDERIZER IN IT?

*Gabby asks: I've seen papaya extract and bromelain listed as ingredients in both hair products and meat tenderizers. What's the story here? Is my hair going to get softer, as meat does when I tenderize it? Or are these ingredients going to break down and damage my hair?*

Lots of shampoos and conditioners contain papaya extract: Aussie and Ojon are just a couple of examples. But that doesn't mean they'll tenderize your hair. To help you understand why, we'll explain the secret superpower of papaya.

## PAPAYA EXTRACT AND PAPAIN

Papaya extract is essentially fruit juice diluted in a solvent like propylene glycol or water and alcohol. Small amounts of this extract in hair care products have no effect. But papain, an enzyme present in fresh papaya, does have some interesting properties. It belongs to a class of chemicals known as proteases, which are able to break down certain kinds of proteins.

Papain is typically made by collecting the milky latex from the fruit of the papaya tree and letting it dry. The purified enzyme can be supplied as a powder or a liquid. The mode of action of papain, for those of you interested in such things, is enzymatic degradation of peptide bonds by deprotonation. In other words, it's your standard nucleophilic attack on the carbonyl carbon of a peptide backbone. All this means is that papain is able to break down the kind of protein of which meat is made. That explains its tenderizing properties.

## PAPAIN AND HAIR

While papain can break down the kind of protein found in meat and muscle tissue, it has little effect on hair because it's made of an even tougher protein called keratin. While there has been some unpublished research investigating the effect of papain as a depilatory or hair relaxer, we can't find any reference to hair being damaged by papaya extract.

## THE BOTTOM LINE

Don't be worried that your hair will be tenderized by your favorite papaya shampoo or conditioner like Maya Papaya Leave-in Conditioner, Tigi S Factor Papaya Leave-in Moisture Spray or Formula's Ecoly Papaya Dry Hair Shampoo. It won't.

**Bonus fact:** Papaya extract can allegedly be used to break down the proteins in bug venom and can therefore speed the healing of certain insect bites. By the way, bromelain is a similar enzyme that comes from pineapples.

# DOES THE MOON CAUSE BAD HAIR DAYS?

*Linda's long-hair lunacy: In the last few years, I have had many friends discuss which phase of the moon is the best for a haircut. Supposedly, your haircut will last longer depending on the cycle. I'm a skeptic, but please enlighten me.*

While there's no direct research proving this point one way or the other, there are a few studies that *may* suggest there's actually some science behind your friends' seemingly bizarre contention.

## THE FULL MOON EFFECT

The idea that the full moon causes people to act crazy has been discredited, but there is at least one study suggesting that the phase of the moon has an impact on certain physiological attributes. We could only find a single study on this and we're curious if the research properly isolated variables because it's pretty much impossible to take the moon effect out of the equation (unless the research is conducted on another planet). Plus, since it is just a single study, we'd want to see some corroborative research before totally buying into this.

But according to the article, "The Lunar Cycle: Effects on Human and Animal Behavior and Physiology" from the Polish Academy of Sciences, the moon does have an effect on certain metabolic processes in animals and humans. For example, the lunar cycle may cause hormonal changes in insects, variations in melatonin levels in birds and taste sensitivity in lab rats. The article posits that the gravitational pull of the moon could be triggering the release of neurohormones, which is the cause of these effects. While the mechanism is unknown, the researchers believe this is an area worth additional study. This seems highly dubious, as the amount of gravitational pull on individual people is extremely low and it isn't affected by whether there is a full moon or not. A half-lit moon pulls on you just as much as a full moon.

## MELATONIN AND THE MANE

The second piece of the puzzle is an article titled "Melatonin and the Hair Follicle," which explains that melatonin has long been known to modulate hair growth (as well as pigmentation and/or molting in many species). Apparently, this is due to its activity as a neuroendocrine regulator, but precisely how it affects the hair follicle is not fully understood. Unspecific melatonin binding sites have been identified in animals such as goats and mice, but scientists don't know the specific binding interaction for humans. This paper focuses on recent discoveries on this interaction.

So, we found one study linking melatonin production to phases of the moon and another showing that melatonin levels influence hair growth. Taken together, these studies suggest that there may be a plausible mechanism for the phase of the moon affecting hair growth. So, theoretically, if you get your hair cut at one point during the lunar cycle, it may grow back more quickly than at another time.

## THE BOTTOM LINE

We're far from convinced by these two studies. The gravitational effect of the moon is too minimal to have an impact on hair. But perhaps future research will shed more (moon) light on this intriguing question. Scientists always love to be proven wrong. It's how we learn.

# CAN MY HAIR SPRAY CONTAINER EXPLODE?

*Susan's sizzling science question:* I know some cosmetics, especially aerosols, come with recommended storage temperatures. Since I live in Texas and the temperature inside a closed vehicle can reach up to 200 degrees Fahrenheit, I was wondering if most cosmetic formulas were thermally stable enough to spend a few days in transit without alteration. Also, since most aerosols warn consumers not to store them at temperatures above 120 degrees Fahrenheit, I was wondering if there had been any incidents of these things exploding in the back of a UPS truck?

Heat can certainly have a detrimental effect on product quality, but there's not too much cause for concern because all reputable cosmetic companies test their products at elevated temperatures.

## COSMETIC STABILITY TESTING

High temperature testing is done for two reasons. The first reason is to predict the long-term stability of the product at normal temperatures. Since the rate of most chemical reactions approximately doubles for every 10-degree Celsius increase in temperature, you can tell if a product will be stable at room temperature for several years by testing it at elevated temperatures for several months.

The second reason for high temperature testing is to screen for exactly the kind of problem you mentioned: To find out if your Ecco Bella Lipstick will turn into "Yuck-a Bella" when it's shipped to Texas (or to Dubai, or just about any place experiencing global warming!). While there's no single, standard, worldwide temperature that is used, in general if a product is stable up to 50 or 54 degrees Celsius (122–129 degrees Fahrenheit) for up to eight weeks, it should be fine under normal shipping conditions. If absolutely necessary, products sensitive to heat (or cold) can be shipped in temperature-controlled vehicles, but this can increase both cost and shipping time.

## EXPLODING HAIRSPRAY?

While we've never personally heard of any cans exploding in transit, it's certainly not impossible. In the United States, the Department of Transportation dictates what requirements cans have to meet to be shipped safely. The rule is that if the pressure in an aerosol can exceeds 180 to 200 pounds per square inch at 130 degrees Fahrenheit, then a special heavy-duty can must be used to ensure that it won't explode.

## THE BOTTOM LINE

It's unlikely that any of your cosmetics will be exposed to temperatures high enough to cause damage to the product—or to explode!

# 7 REASONS TO AVOID HOME ELECTROLYSIS

Electrolysis is a process that involves inserting the tip of a metal stylus into your hair follicle; the stylus shoots a mild electric current through your skin to destroy the root of the hair. You then remove the hair from the follicle with tweezers and, if you're lucky, it never grows back. Even when done professionally, this process can be hard to sit through, but it does eliminate, or at least greatly delay, hair regrowth.

Should you attempt this on your own at home? Scientifically speaking, we think the risks outweigh the benefits.

**1** **The process is difficult and time-consuming**
Since each hair must be individually treated, it can take a *long* time to treat a large area. The more hair you have, the longer the process. That may not be so bad when someone else is doing the work, but it's hard when you have to do it all yourself.

**2** **A greater chance of skin damage**
Since the average person doesn't have the same training, experience and equipment as a professional, you're more likely to damage your follicle. And any kind of damage can leave you with a permanent scar.

**3** **Results may not last as long**
If you're not skilled in the process and you don't destroy the entire root, the hair could grow back. Even if you *do* get the entire root, there's no guarantee that the hair won't come back. According to the FDA's Anthony Watson, "the stimulus for hair growth in an area is never permanently removed. For instance, you can't control hormonal changes that cause new growth. Most people would probably define permanent as 'never comes back,' but from a medical standpoint that may not be practical."

###  Increased side effects

By doing electrolysis yourself, you may see a greater incidence of redness and swelling than with professional treatment. It's a temporary effect, but it's unpleasant nonetheless.

###  Heightened pain level

Our personal favorite. Even though neither method uses a dangerously high level of electricity, some people find home electrolysis more painful than professional treatment.

###  More expensive

When you consider your time, plus the equipment and additional supplies you'll need to buy, home treatment may not be as cheap as you think. But, then again, professional treatments are expensive, too.

### 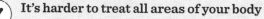 It's harder to treat all areas of your body

Remember that it's hard to reach some of the areas you'll want to treat—either because you're looking at yourself backwards in the mirror or because you're not using your dominant hand. The American Medical Association's Committee on Cutaneous Health and Cosmetics says the success of electrolysis self-treatment depends largely on the condition of the hair and skin, the equipment and the level of skill you've developed. The committee recommends limiting self-treatment to readily accessible areas, such as the lower parts of the arms and legs.

# PART II

# SKIN

# 4 SKIN TREATMENTS—FROM SILLY TO SUBLIME

People have tried innumerable ways to get great-looking skin, but few can tell whether these really work. Here we discuss various treatments and determine if they help your skin in any way. If you're looking for a magic way to get wrinkle-free skin, you won't find it in this chapter (because it doesn't exist yet). But you will find a suprising way to make skin look brighter and younger, learn how to properly apply sunscreen and how to use duct tape to get rid of warts.

# THE BEST SKIN MOISTURIZING OILS IN THE WORLD

**Pamela ponders:** *Since the weather is getting drier, I've decided to look for some treatments to keep my cuticles from drying out. I've noticed that a lot of the products include very similar ingredients, like jojoba oil, apricot kernel oil, shea butter and, in particular, sweet almond oil and lavender oil. Do these ingredients really help to moisturize and what exactly do they do? I've noticed a lot of body care products emphasize shea butter. I've also noticed some body lotions have coconut oil in them. Is this another beneficial ingredient?*

All the oils you mentioned can moisturize skin, but they're not the *best* moisturizers. Which *are* the best, you ask?

## HOW OILS MOISTURIZE

Moisture evaporates from your skin by slipping though tiny cracks and fissures. Oils form a barrier layer on top of the skin that prevents the water molecules from escaping. It's all about stopping evaporation! This property is called occlusivity and it's measured by a rating called transepidermal water loss, or TEWL (pronounced "tool"). The TEWL value has been measured for various oils, and the ones that have the highest rating (those that stop the most water from escaping your skin) are as listed here.

### Top five moisturizing oils (according to cosmetics science)

1. Petroleum jelly (at a concentration of 5%, reduces TEWL by more than 98%)
2. Lanolin
3. Mineral oil
4. Dimethicone (a type of silicone)
5. Others, including other oils (like coconut), fatty alcohols and waxes

## THE BOTTOM LINE

Some of the other oils you mention are still beneficial—they can make skin feel softer and smoother. But if you really want to keep your skin and cuticles moist, you need to reduce evaporation with one of these top five.

# THREE REASONS WHY MOISTURIZERS FOR THE HANDS AND FACE SHOULD BE DIFFERENT

**Kay's question:** *Is there a difference between moisturizers for your hands and for your face? Also, is there a reason to use specially formulated antiwrinkle creams rather than ordinary moisturizers that you would use on your hands?*

This is one of those cases where there really is some science behind the marketing hype. Here's why facial lotions should be different than hand lotions:

**1** **Skin on the hands and face is different.**
Skin is very thin on your face and thicker on your hands. Also, your hands don't (usually) develop acne or blackheads. Therefore, they need to be treated differently.

**2** **Drying conditions are different for the hands and face.**
You may wash your hands in harsh soap many times a day; you may wash your face only once or twice a day with a gentle cleanser. Hands are in and out of dishwater or laundry water; your face is not. The cumulative effect is that your hands can be much dryer, even cracked and bleeding, and therefore they need stronger moisturization.

**3** **The hands and face have different cosmetic needs.**
You might want to tighten the little crow's-feet wrinkles around your eyes, but this isn't the case on your hands.

## THE BOTTOM LINE

For the reasons cited above and more, you need to use products designed to suit your skin's different needs. Hand lotions should be heavier barrier creams to protect hands from harsh conditions. Facial moisturizers should be lightweight, noncomedogenic and may have film-forming agents that tighten skin to help reduce the appearance of fine lines and wrinkles. While hand and face products may share some of the same basic ingredients, the functions they need to perform are significantly different. Using the right product on the right skin will give you better results.

# DO PORE STRIPS REALLY WORK?

*Andrea asks:* What can you tell me about Bioré-type pore strips? It's strangely fascinating seeing all the crap that comes off on the strips, but is this just a quick fix that will actually make things worse in the long run?

A pore strip, like the one made by Bioré, is a very dramatic way to clean your pores. It works by adhering to your skin so tightly that when you pull it off it also pulls out the oily, dirty gunk that is clogging your pores.

## PORE STRIPS REALLY WORK

The cool thing is that you can actually see the pore poop stuck to the strip after you take it off. The first time the Beauty Brains evaluators tried this product, they sat staring transfixed at the forest of tiny nasal pore discharge dotting the landscape of the freshly spent pore strip. Some whiteheads were barely visible to the naked eye; other blackheads were ominously thick and dark. We still get shivers just thinking about it.

Even if you don't feel you need them, we recommend trying pore strips as an experiment just so you can see for yourself.

## THE PROBLEM WITH PORE STRIPS

When used correctly, pore strips can be a powerful weapon in your battle against blackheads. But don't use them too often because they can irritate your skin. Three times per week max. Any more than that and you risk damaging your skin. You should heed the warnings on the box about not using them on any area other than the nose and not to use them over inflamed, swollen, sunburned or excessively dry skin. If you use pore strips too often, they can actually irritate your skin and trigger more breakouts.

# DOES RETIN-A ELIMINATE WRINKLES?

*Belinda begs:* I've read that Retin-A helps get rid of wrinkles. True or false?

Retin-A is the brand name of a prescription drug called Tretinoin, which is a derivative of vitamin A. In 1971, the FDA approved the topical application of Tretinoin to treat acne and sun-damaged skin. This drug works by irritating the skin, which triggers the basal layer to produce fresh skin cells, thus increasing cell turnover. (Mmmm, turnover!) As new cells more rapidly replace the old ones, the skin takes on a younger, smoother appearance. So it does work, but there are a few issues of which you should be aware.

### Six things you need to know about Retin-A

1. It is a prescription drug, so you can only get it from your doctor.

2. It doesn't work overnight. Wrinkles start to decrease or disappear after three to six months.

3. Some of the drug is absorbed into the body and may cause problems with pregnancy.

4. It can be so irritating that it burns and causes redness.

5. While it does help reduce wrinkles, that doesn't mean it gets rid of *all* your wrinkles. As they say, results will vary.

6. Sun protection should always be worn while using Retin-A because the drug can lead to severe burns.

## THE BOTTOM LINE

Unlike so many wrinkle creams, this drug has been proven to really do something (despite the issues cited above). And don't fall for the claims of other products that are just regular cosmetics with vitamin A derivatives.

# AN INEXPENSIVE, NATURAL WRINKLE REMOVER FROM THE DAIRY CASE

*Mandy's got milk:* I am fifty-four years young and when I was twenty-two I was told to put buttermilk on my face to get rid of wrinkles. I've been using it ever since, and there is no question that my skin looks much younger than that of other women my age. I have also stayed out of the sun and don't smoke, and today I also use pricey beauty products like ReVive and Origins. Do you think it's buttermilk that's keeping my skin wrinkle-free?

Could buttermilk be responsible for your youthful appearance? Mmmmmmaybe. But doubtful. Here's why.

## WHAT THE HECK IS BUTTERMILK, ANYWAY?

For those of you who aren't up to speed on your dairy products, buttermilk is a thickened, sour type of milk that is made by adding lactococcus lactis bacteria to regular milk. The bacteria cause fermentation, which changes the milk sugar (aka lactose) into lactic acid. Sound familiar? It should! Lactic acid is an alpha hydroxy acid (or AHA), the same chemical that's used in anti-aging lotions to exfoliate your skin. Unfortunately, it doesn't look like buttermilk is any better than lotions you can buy.

## WHY ISN'T BUTTERMILK BETTER?

Milk contains 4–6 percent lactose. When it's converted to buttermilk, you end up with about 3 or 4 percent lactic acid. Lactic acid skin creams contain about 12 percent lactic acid—about three times as much as buttermilk. So, while it's theoretically possible that buttermilk could be helping, you'd probably see more benefit from a relatively inexpensive lactic acid cream like Lac-hydrin.

## SO, IF IT'S NOT THE BUTTERMILK, WHY DOES YOUR SKIN LOOK GOOD?

There could be several other reasons your skin looks so good. First, genetics plays a large role in the health of your skin. It might also be your healthy lifestyle. By staying out of the sun and not smoking, you've avoided two of the major causes of premature aging. Finally, you said that you're using other beauty products, like Revive and Origins, along with the buttermilk. If any of these products contain sunscreen, that could be preventing your skin from aging, too.

## THE BOTTOM LINE

While there is some lactic acid in buttermilk that could help your skin, traditional lactic acid skin creams have a much higher level and will work better. There's nothing wrong with using buttermilk, but there's no proof that it's providing much extra benefit.

# ARE ORAL SUPPLEMENTS GOOD FOR YOUR SKIN?

**Cheong asks:** *Do oral skin supplements like Imedeen really work? I do believe that you are what you eat, and a healthy diet does help your skin, but can taking things like collagen or bird's nest soup or ginseng really give you better skin?*

We get these questions all the time, asking if various food supplements are going to help skin, hair, weight loss and even longevity.

## SUPPLEMENTS ARE UNREGULATED... THAT'S BAD

The claims on some of these things are so wild it seems that just popping a pill every day should fix every problem you've got. Of course, this is nonsense. Remember, food and health supplements are *not regulated*. They can say *anything* they want, even if it is a *lie*, and no one will likely do anything about it. So, when it comes to supplements, the first reaction for every Beauty Brainiac should be one of skepticism.

## WHAT'S IMEDEEN'S STORY?

So, what about Imedeen? Imedeen is basically a skincare supplement that includes proteins, polysaccharides, vitamin C and other "free radical scavengers." According to the company...

*Imedeen Time Perfection is state-of-the-art skincare based on natural ingredients that are scientifically documented to visibly reduce signs of aging from within and to help defend against new signs of aging from forming.*

And after just two to three months of use, you are supposed to see results. Hope in a bottle is finally here! Yeah, right. Although, in the event that you don't notice anything after a month of use, they include this disclaimer:

*As with any nutritional supplement, the response will vary from person to person, and depends on skin condition, general health, diet, environment and other factors.*

This basically means that if it doesn't work for you, then there must be something wrong with *you*, not with the product.

First, the notion that what you eat affects the condition of your skin may make sense but few, if any, studies have shown any link between diet and skin condition. Unless you are malnourished, there will not be any substantial difference in your skin. It's highly unlikely that using this supplement will have any noticeable effect.

## IMEDEEN MAKES A LOT OF STRONG CLAIMS

Next, let's look at some of the company's specific claims for this supplement.

1. Instantly begins to neutralize the skin-degrading processes
2. Significantly improves the skin's moisture balance
3. Visibly reduces the appearance of fine lines and wrinkles
4. Diminishes the visibility of dilated capillaries and age spots
5. Leaves the skin with a brighter, more youthful and even complexion
6. Helps shield and defend the vital structural elements of the skin against future degradation

## BUT THERE'S VERY LITTLE SUPPORTIVE DATA

What do these claims really mean? The first claim sounds compelling, but it doesn't mean all that much. "Instantly begins"? Why doesn't it "instantly neutralize"? And notice how the marketing gurus don't spell out what the "skin-degrading processes" are? What could they possibly mean? They are hoping you'll come up with something that you think is "skin-degrading" and believe that this stuff stops it.

The second claim doesn't make much sense, either. What is the "skin's moisture balance"? The only factors that can affect this are the condition of your skin and environmental factors, like temperature and humidity.

What about the rest of the claims? Reduces fine lines and wrinkles? These claims come from the company's scientific data. But a study that the marketers reference as proof clearly concludes that after three months there are "no significant effects detected." It is only after *nine more months* of an uncontrolled study that the Imedeen shows any effect. Unfortunately, with an uncontrolled study, there is no way to tell what caused the positive results the researchers observed. This is extremely weak data!

The sixth and final claim also is pretty worthless. How do you prove that a product can "shield and defend" against future skin damage? You can't! What a bunch of marketing gobbledygook.

The most outrageous part of this supplement is how much it costs. According to our friends at beauty.com, a box of Imedeen contains sixty tablets (one month of treatment) and costs $70. So you'll have to buy $210 worth of supplements to see any effect, if there is any effect. In fact, since Imedeen's own study says it'll take nine months to see a benefit, that will set you back a whopping $630! Is that worth it to you?

## THE BOTTOM LINE

Imedeen has some slick marketing and even a couple of "studies" to back up its claims. But with the prices the company charges, the weakness of their data and the fact that you'll still have to apply sunscreen and moisturizer, this doesn't seem to us like a smart purchase at all. You'd be better off saving your money for plastic surgery. And as far as collagen, bird's nest soup or ginseng giving you better skin…we don't think so.

# IS AN ASPIRIN MASK GOOD FOR SKIN?

*Ivy asks about aspirin: What's the deal with aspirin masks? The mask is prepared by crushing four aspirins and mixing them with a bit of water to create a paste. Then it's smeared over your face. What is it supposed to do?*

Aspirin masks seem to be all the rage these days, but we can't find any evidence that they're worth the effort. Here's why.

## WHAT IS ASPIRIN?

The active ingredient in aspirin is the drug called acetylsalicylic acid. After you swallow an aspirin tablet, it travels to your small intestine where this ingredient is broken down to create salicylic acid. Salicylic acid, or sal acid as it's sometimes called, is the form of the drug that actually reduces pain, fever and so on.

Now, sal acid also belongs to the class of chemicals known as beta hydroxy acids, or BHAs. BHAs are similar to AHAs (alpha hydroxy acids). Both BHAs and AHAs are known for their ability to help slough off dead skin cells when applied topically. Are you beginning to see the connection between aspirin and facial masks?

## WHY ASPIRIN ISN'T GOOD FOR YOUR SKIN

In theory, crushing aspirin tablets and rubbing them on your face *could* be beneficial because you're delivering a skin-smoothing BHA, right? Well, not exactly.

You're really delivering acetylsalicylic acid to the skin—*not* salicylic acid, which is the active BHA. And just rubbing the acetyl version on your skin won't make it convert to the sal acid version. OK, maybe *some* of the acid is present in the sal version, but it certainly isn't an optimized dose.

## THE BOTTOM LINE

Putting crushed aspirin on your face might have *some* benefit, but if you really want a skin-smoothing BHA treatment, just buy one of the many sal acid products on the market. In this case, the home remedy doesn't appear as effective as the chemist-made one.

# A SAFE WAY TO MAKE YOUR SKIN LOOK BRIGHTER AND YOUNGER

*Margaret wants to know:* *I use Definity products and they work well for me, but are all the products basically the same? And I've heard they contain hydroquinone. Is that safe?*

According to P&G, which makes Definity, it "fights what ages you most: discoloration, dullness, brown spots, and wrinkles." The fighting wrinkles stuff is pretty standard in beauty creams. If you're hydrating the skin (especially if you're using a film-forming agent that helps hide fine lines), you can support antiwrinkle claims. The interesting aspect of Definity is that it claims to make the skin more luminous because it gets rid of darkness and dullness.

## HOW DOES DEFINITY MAKE SKIN LUMINOUS?

Skin-lightening claims like these normally involve hydroquinone, a skin-bleaching agent that's come under fire for safety reasons. Fortunately, Definity doesn't contain hydroquinone. Instead, it uses N-acetyl glucosamine, a chemical that inhibits glyco-sylation of pro-tyrosinase. (Relax: That just means it prevents the kind of chemical reactions that make liver spots and freckles.) N-acetyl glucosamine (or NAG as it's known) is not as effective as hydroquinone, but it's safer to use.

Sound too good to be true? Check out the multiple clinical test results that show that glucosamine effectively prevents dark age spots. And if dark spots are reduced, skin will look lighter and more luminous.

Of course, the question is, how *much* improvement will you really see? The only way to tell for sure is to try the product. But at least Olay has done its homework and formulated a product line that's based on science, not snake oil.

## THE DEFINITY LINE

There are six Definity products altogether: Definity Foaming Moisturizer, Foaming Moisturizer with UV absorber, Correcting Protective Lotion, Intense Hydrating Cream, Illuminating Cream Cleanser, and Pore Redefining Scrub.

Why six products? Is it because P&G is satanically trying to remind you of 666, the mark of the beast? Oh, wait, that's a myth; P&G is not run by satanists. So there must be another reason that it would offer six different products. Actually, we can think of three reasons and they all boil down to trying to catch the attention of you, the shopper.

**1** **Providing solutions to multiple skin care problems**
Four of the products are moisturizers; two of those contain a UV absorber. The other two products are cleansers. By offering different benefits across the product line, Olay appeals to women seeking solutions to different skin care problems.

**2** **Offering similar benefits in different formats**
If you like to put on a heavier moisturizer at night, you can use the Intense Hydrating Cream. If you prefer a lighter product in the morning, you can use the Foaming Moisturizer. By offering similar products in different formats, they appeal to a broader audience.

**3** **Creating a stronger shelf presence**
Let's face it, cosmetics companies are in business to sell products. To sell products they have to make them available to consumers, which means getting their products onto store shelves. And the more products on the shelf, the easier it is for consumers to find them. This is a strategy known as "brand blocking." Companies put as many of their products together on a shelf as possible to create a stronger impression. So one of the reasons there are six different Definity products is that it makes good business sense.

OK, to be fair to Olay, they don't say that you have to use all six products. They recommend using a cleanser, a moisturizer and a sunscreen moisturizer. But wait. That means you're using two moisturizers: One Protects and Corrects and the other Perfects and Deflects. Or is that Detects and Reflects? Connects and Rejects? Arrrrrh! This is confusing!

## THE BOTTOM LINE

Definity does contain an ingredient proven to lighten skin. Of course, that doesn't guarantee that you'll notice a difference yourself. It's a bit expensive at $22 for 1.7 ounces, but at least its claims are based on real science. If you're curious, pick a Definity moisturizer and cleanser that you like and give them a try. If you don't notice a difference after a few weeks, don't buy them again.

# WHAT'S THE RIGHT WAY TO APPLY SUNSCREEN?

*Kim's query:* My question is about sunscreen: On the bottle, it says to apply fifteen to thirty minutes before sun exposure so the product can be absorbed. Say I apply sunscreen to my hands, wait half an hour, then wash them. Will the skin on my hands still be protected from the sun? Or do I need to apply again, and wait another thirty minutes?

First of all, if you're washing off the sunscreen you've already put on, it doesn't matter if you wait the thirty minutes or not. You've got to leave it on or it won't work. But if you're just concerned about protecting your hands, we wouldn't worry too much. You can apply sunscreen to your hands and then just carefully wash the palms so they don't feel greasy. That way the backs of your hands will be protected and there's little chance that your palms will get enough sun to cause a problem. But if you're still worried about it, you could always wear gloves at the beach, as the Left Brain does!

Still confused about how to apply sunscreen? Here's what the American Academy of Dermatologists recommends.

### Three simple steps to safer sun protection

1. **Put on plenty:** An ounce or so (about a shot glass full) should about do it for the average person.

2. **Soak it up:** For maximum protection, wait for it to soak in before (15–30 minutes) frolicking in the sun.

3. **Frequent reapplication:** Reapply often, at least every 2 hours.

Why is this last item so important? First, because the UV-absorbing molecules can wear out over time so your protection level drops off. Second, because sweating, swimming and towel-drying can remove sunscreen from your skin's surface. Do you really have to put more on after only 2 hours? Apparently, yes. Studies have shown that people who wait 2½ hours instead of 2, have a five times greater chance of burning.

Yes, this means you might go through an entire bottle of sunscreen during a day at the beach. But that's still cheaper than a visit to your friendly neighborhood dermatologist to have a spot of melanoma removed!

# HOW CAN YOU TELL IF YOUR SUNSCREEN HAS GONE BAD?

*Catherine's concerned about sunscreen efficacy: I've heard that when sunscreen/sunblock separates, it's no longer good, and that shaking it up to remix it is basically wasted effort and applying it will do no good at all. Is this true? Can sunscreen go bad?*

Sunscreen formulations are very sensitive creatures. Most UV absorbers are oil-soluble, which means they have to be carefully emulsified to form stable mixtures with water. If the oil and water in the formula are not properly coupled together, the whole formula can go to hell pretty quickly. Here are three warning signs that your sunscreen has gone sour.

**1 Weird consistency**
The consistency of the product has changed over time and now it's too thick or too thin to spread properly. The spreadability of sunscreens is crucial to proper application and coverage. If it doesn't spread right, it won't work right.

**2 Crystallization**
The active ingredient has crystallized out, making the lotion feel gritty. When this happens, the product is completely worthless. You can't fix that by shaking it.

**3 Separation**
The product has separated into two different layers. Also, not good. At worst, the active ingredient will seep into the oil phase and shaking it may or may not resuspend it properly. At best, the water resistance of the product may be compromised and it will wash off too easily. Either way, it's really not worth using. Go buy a fresh bottle.

## THE BOTTOM LINE

Given the importance of good UV protection, don't take chances with a bottle of sunscreen that you think may have gone bad. Most manufacturers should gladly refund your money or offer you a replacement if you have a problem.

# CURE WARTS WITH DUCT TAPE

Here's a great tip for the do-it-yourself crowd: Duct tape can cure warts!

Yes, it's true, according to Anthony J. Mancini, MD, an associate professor at Northwestern University's School of Medicine and the head of pediatric dermatology at Children's Memorial Hospital in Chicago. Dr. Mancini says he uses duct tape as an inexpensive and relatively painless way to treat warts. He has his patients apply the duct tape over the wart, leave it on for about a week, remove the tape, and then file the wart with an emery board. It's that easy.

But how can such a simple household item treat a sustained viral infection?

No one knows, at least not for sure. But theoretically the tape could be debriding, or stripping the dead skin from the wart and carrying the wart virus along with it. That's kind of how other wart therapies work (like the Compound W or Kryoderm freezing technique). Another possible mechanism is that occluding skin with duct tape somehow triggers the patient's immune system to fight the virus. There's no solid data to support this theory, but doctors do use immunotherapy against warts in some patients.

# CAN SKIN CREAMS CAUSE CANCER?

**Lorraine asks:** *Many skin creams say that they will increase cell production. How do they make sure that doesn't include cancer cells that may be dormant in the body?*

If skin creams really did affect cell production, cancer could be a huge problem. So why haven't we seen a drastic increase in skin cancer? You can probably guess the answer.

## SKIN CREAMS DO NOT INCREASE CELL PRODUCTION

No matter how a personal care product is marketed, unless it is an illegal drug it will not have any effect on cell metabolism. According to the definitions set up by the FDA (the U.S. government agency that oversees cosmetic and drug regulations), cosmetics are articles intended to be rubbed, poured, sprinkled, or sprayed on, introduced into, or otherwise applied to the human body for cleansing, beautifying, promoting attractiveness or altering the appearance.

The FDA defines a drug as:

*articles (other than food) intended to affect the structure or any function of the body of man or other animals.*

Basically, cosmetics are products that are used to temporarily change the appearance of your body. Products that affect the body's metabolism (such as by increasing cell production) are drugs, which require a lot more rigorous testing.

## ARE COSMETIC COMPANIES LYING?

In general, cosmetic companies are not explicitly lying. There are some rogue companies that do, but that is a small minority in the cosmetics industry. More common are companies that word claims in such a way that they trick you into believing something is true even when they don't say it directly.

For example, you are under the impression that the skin cream you are using will "increase cell production." But unless you purchased it from a disreputable company, it probably doesn't actually claim to increase cell production. Look at the exact wording of the claim. You will likely find one of the following.

**1** **"Helps stimulate skin cell production."**
By using the word *helps*, the company isn't lying outright because applying anything to skin could "help" stimulate cell production. As long as it is vague about what *helping* means, it's considered OK.

**2** **"With [ingredient] shown to increase cell production."**
Often a claim is worded so that it refers to an ingredient shown to stimulate cell production in laboratory tests. It's easy to show an ingredient affecting cell growth in a lab, but it's much more difficult to get it to work on actual skin. By claiming that a product "with" a certain ingredient can stimulate cell growth, the company isn't specifically saying the product causes cell growth, but that is the impression you might get.

## THE BOTTOM LINE

Don't worry; skin creams are not going to cause outbreaks of cancer. They don't really affect cell growth. Claims made by cosmetics companies are often written in a way that is not exactly a lie, but is designed to trick you into believing something that they aren't actually saying. When you see a fantastic claim on a bottle, think about what the words mean precisely as written. Then you might be able to see through the trick.

# WHY CAN'T SUNSCREEN BE MADE TO LAST LONGER?

**Kelly asks:** *Really, why can't sunscreen stay on? Is there any possibility of making a sunscreen that works from the inside, such as in pill form, or a lotion/spray that will actually be absorbed into cells, like a spray tan?*

Of all the things you can do to keep young-looking skin, applying sunscreen daily is perhaps the most effective and important. It's unfortunate that it is so inconvenient.

## LONG-LASTING SUNSCREEN

There are a few reasons sunscreen doesn't stay on longer, and they all involve water. Some sunscreens like Ensulizole and Mexoryl SX are soluble in water so they easily come off when exposed to water. Most other sunscreens, like oxybenzone, octyl methoxycinnamate or titanium dioxde, are not water-soluble, but they will also come off, just not as quickly.

Avoiding water completely will not help because sunscreen is slowly removed from the skin when you perspire. The water and salt that you naturally produce will disrupt the sunscreen film and leave parts of your skin unprotected.

Even if scientists could figure out a way to create sunscreens that stay on skin like Krazy Glue, they would still have a limited duration because the outer layer of your skin is constantly being shed and chemical sunscreens naturally stop working after they've been exposed to enough UV radiation.

All this means is that no matter which sunscreen you use, you should reapply it at least every 2 hours.

## INSIDE OUT

The idea of taking a sunscreen pill is an appealing one and something scientists continue to work on.

Some compounds have been shown to have a UV-blocking effect when eaten. According to a study published in the March 2003 issue of the *International Journal for Vitamin and Nutrition Research*, the ingredient lycopene, which is found in tomato paste, has been shown to provide some protection. Also carotenoids, found in sweet potatoes, carrots, apricots and squash, have some UV-protective effects. Unfortunately, these foods do not provide nearly enough protection. In the future, scientists may develop better-working, ingestible sunscreens, but until they do, you'd better keep slathering on the traditional stuff.

## A SPRAY THAT IS ABSORBED INTO THE SKIN

A spray sunscreen that is absorbed into the skin would make an interesting product, but not one that scientists have been able to create thus far. It's not certain whether this would even be a good idea because some evidence suggests that if sunscreens like titanium dioxide or zinc oxide get into the body, they can build up and cause problems. Incidentally, sunless tanners do not actually penetrate the skin. They react with skin surface proteins to create the brown color.

## THE BOTTOM LINE

Sunscreen is one of the best cosmetics you can use to keep your skin looking young and wrinkle-free. All sunscreens will wash or wear off, so you should reapply frequently when you're out in the sun. Ingestible products may be the future of sunscreens, but they just are not effective enough yet.

# DOES GLYCERIN DRY OUT SKIN?

*Frances is befuddled:* *Is it true that glycerin moisturizes the surface of the skin, but extracts the moisture from deeper levels, causing dryness beneath?*

Ever wonder where rumors like these get started? We imagine they start with somebody's mom, who heard it from one of her friends, who heard it from her stylist. We doubt information about cosmetic chemicals ever starts with cosmetics scientists.

## WHAT IS GLYCERIN?

Let's first look at what it is. Glycerin (or glycerol) is a colorless, odorless, liquid compound that is used in numerous personal care and pharmaceutical applications. It has a sweet taste, is sticky and is a natural by-product of the soap-making process.

## WHY IS IT USED IN SKIN PRODUCTS?

Cosmetics chemists use glycerin in beauty products for the skin because it is an excellent moisturizing ingredient. It will attract and hold water, keeping skin soft and smooth without an itchy feeling. The only drawback to glycerin is that it can make your skin feel sticky if you use too much of it.

## DOES IT EXTRACT MOISTURE FROM DEEPER LEVELS?

Glycerin does attract water from anywhere, but most of that water is pulled from either the air or the skin cream. There is a potential for glycerin to extract too much moisture from the deeper layers of skin and cause dryness or dehydration of skin; however, this only happens with very high concentrations of glycerin. If *water* is the first ingredient on the formula list, you won't have this problem. Just avoid using pure glycerin as a hand treatment and you'll be OK.

## THE BOTTOM LINE

Glycerin is one of the best moisturizing ingredients that cosmetics chemists have found. It makes skin look and feel better and as long as you don't use too much, it is a perfectly safe ingredient to use.

# WHAT IS GALVANIC STIMULATION AND DOES IT DO ANYTHING FOR SKIN?

*Alina asks:* What exactly does "galvanic stimulation" (used in facials) do for the skin?

Galvanic stimulation is one of those terms that sounds highly technical and impressive, but when you look at the available research, you realize that it is less science than it is unfounded hope.

## WHAT IS GALVANIC STIMULATION?

Galvanic stimulation refers to a form of electrotherapy using a device that can create an electrical charge that is either positive or negative. During the treatment, a gel containing negatively charged surfactants is applied to your skin. The device is then rubbed on the skin and the negative ions it creates are supposed to enhance the penetration of the negatively charged gel. Like repels like, remember?

Next, the excess gel is removed and a second, positively charged gel, containing all kinds of nutritious ingredients, is applied. The device is switched to the positive ion setting and again massaged on the skin. This time, the positive charges are supposed to help the gel ingredients penetrate more deeply and improve your skin tone.

## DOES IT WORK?

We went through all the medical literature published in the last few decades and could find no studies that supported claims that galvanic stimulation enhances the skin. It has been used to help with the management of pain stemming from injuries and it could help with wound healing, although the evidence for these claims is minimal at best. However, there is no evidence that it works to promote the penetration of skin ingredients. Galvanic stimulation might make for a good story, but that doesn't mean it works.

The problem with galvanic stimulation is that the forces involved are not strong enough to overcome the skin barrier. Even if there was a slight repellant effect, this wouldn't make much difference when it came to penetration. The cosmetic-ingredient molecules are just not small enough to penetrate deeply into skin.

## WHY DO PEOPLE SAY THEIR SKIN LOOKS BETTER AFTER TREATMENT?

While there is no scientific evidence that galvanic stimulation has any effect on skin appearance, you'll see plenty of testimonials touting its benefits from satisfied customers. There are two explanations for this. First, the mere act of massaging skin for a few minutes can change the way skin looks. It stimulates blood flow and can help exaggerate the effect of the gels. Second, the people getting the treatment want it to work and are more inclined to believe that their skin looks better. No one wants to think they wasted more than $150 for a treatment that didn't work.

## THE BOTTOM LINE

Galvanic stimulation is an unproven treatment that most likely will not have any long-term benefit for your skin. If you want great-looking skin, skip the galvanic treatment and give yourself an at-home facial. The experience may not be as relaxing, but the results on your skin will be just as good and you'll save a lot of money.

# DOES SNAKE VENOM WORK AS WELL AS BOTOX?

*Sharon says:* A peptide called Syn-ake is being touted for relaxing deep forehead wrinkles. Does it really work? Isn't there some potential for the chemical to travel and cause the eye area to sag? Any restrictions on using this?

You've got to hand it to cosmetic-product marketers. They see that a highly poisonous toxin like Botox is wildly popular as an anti-aging treatment, so they figure people might want to try other poisonous ingredients, too. That led them to snake venom and the development of Syn-ake.

Syn-ake is an antiwrinkle material based on a synthetic tripeptide that "mimics" the effects of a peptide found in the venom of the temple viper snake. It was developed by Pentapharm Ltd., a Swiss-based chemical company—reportedly, the largest snake breeders and keepers in the world.

## WHAT DOES SYN-AKE DO?

According to the company literature, Syn-ake acts in a manner similar to a peptide in snake venom. It supposedly blocks some receptors, relaxes the muscles and smoothes out your wrinkles. Relaxation of muscles is also how Botox works.

## DOES IT WORK?

According to company literature, data from two studies are shown. One study demonstrates that Syn-ake reduces muscle cell contractions in a laboratory test. The second study shows that after twenty-eight days of using a Syn-ake-laced cream, wrinkles shrink up to 52 percent.

That must mean it works, right? Well, not necessarily.

## PROBLEMS WITH THE STUDIES

There are a number of questions about the Syn-ake studies that remain unanswered.

1. What was the placebo to which Syn-ake was compared?
2. Does Syn-ake penetrate to the dermis, where it might possibly have an effect?
3. How does the performance of Syn-ake compare to that of Botox or any other antiwrinkle treatment?
4. How many subjects were tested?
5. Who did the testing and was it blinded?

There are more questions, but the point is that the data are incomplete and not useful for drawing definitive conclusions. A quick search of the medical literature revealed that there were no peer-reviewed studies of this ingredient. With such thin data and such incredible claims, we remain skeptical.

In the sales literature for the Syn-ake peptide, marketers use some language that raises more questions. For example, they say it "mimics the effect" of a peptide found in snake venom. It also says Syn-ake "acts in a manner similar to that of Waglerin 1" (the compound in snake venom shown to block the acetylcholine receptor). *Mimics* and *similar to* are words that marketing companies use to create the impression that two things are related, even when they aren't.

## CAN IT AFFECT YOUR EYES?

If Syn-ake actually performed the way that is implied in your question, then there would be a potential problem with eye sag. If you sweat or water dripped off your forehead, it might get into your eyes. Of course, this would be a minor concern because cosmetics ingredients do not normally travel around on your face once you put them there.

Currently, there are no restrictions on the use of Syn-ake or almost any other anti-aging ingredient in cosmetics. Any ingredient that has been proven to have anything but a superficial cosmetic effect gets regulated as a drug by the FDA (in the United States). Since there is no proof that this ingredient works, there are no official restrictions.

## THE BOTTOM LINE

There is no credible evidence that this material works as well as Botox, no matter how much of it you put on your wrinkles. If you want the effectiveness of Botox, save up your money for Botox. Snake venom creams just will not be as effective. On the plus side, since it probably isn't effective, you also don't have to worry about any potential negative side effects, like causing the eye area to sag.

# ARE EXPENSIVE SELF-TANNERS WORTH THE MONEY?

*Lauren wonders:* My beauty question would have to be this: Is there any difference between all the self-tanners on the market? I know they all feature dihydroxyacetone (DHA) to change skin color, so does it really matter if one costs $30 while one is $7.99? Is it just a matter of branding?

We are always thrilled to see evidence that skepticism is building among beauty-product consumers. This is exactly the kind of question you should be asking about all your products! Time and time again we see that price and performance are not necessarily related. And when it comes to sunless tanners, the story is the same.

## HOW DHA WORKS

First, let's talk about dihydroxyacetone, or DHA. It is a sugar derivative that was discovered in the 1920s. In a formula, it is a clear, colorless ingredient, but when it touches skin, DHA causes a chemical reaction with the surface proteins, which results in a brownish/orange color. The amount of color you get from DHA is directly dependent on how much you put on the skin. Put on a lot, and your skin will resemble the Great Pumpkin. But put on a little, and you get a highly desired, light brown glow. Of all the sunless tanning products available, only those containing DHA are said to be effective by the American Academy of Dermatology. So, if the product is going to work, it's going to have to have DHA.

## FORMULA DIFFERENCES

To see if there is a significant difference between a drugstore brand and an expensive formula, it is helpful to look at their ingredients lists.

Here is the ingredients list of a sunless tanner that runs $37 for eight ounces: water (aqua), dihydroxyacetone, caprylic/capric triglyceride, glycerin, prunus armeniaca kernel oil (apricot), glyceryl stearate, PEG 100 stearate, cetearyl alcohol, cetyl alcohol, sorbitan stearate, dimethicone, aloe barbadensis leaf juice, chamomilla recutita flower extract (matricaria), ceteareth 20, sclerotium gum, butylene glycol, potassium sorbate, phenoxyethanol, sodium bisulfite, fragrance, benzyl salicylate, cinnamal, cinnamyl alcohol, citronellol, coumarin, eugenol, alpha isomethyl ionone, geraniol, hexyl cinnamal, hydroxycitronellal, isoeugenol, butylphenyl methlpropional, linalool, hydroxyisohexyl 3 cyclohexene carboxaldehyde, citric acid, caramel, yellow 6 (CI 15985), red 40 (CI 16035), blue 1 (CI 42090).

Compare that to the ingredients of a sunless tanner that goes for $7 for 7.5 ounces: water, glycerin, aluminum starch octenylsuccinate, C12 15 alkyl benzoate, C13 14 isoparaffin, glyceryl stearate, polyacrylamide, behenyl alcohol, dimethicone, phenyltrimethicone, PFG 100 stearate, tocopheryl acetate, steareth 2, cetyl alcohol, xanthan gum, laureth 7, citric acid, methylparaben, propylparaben, DMDM hydantoin, fragrance, caramel, dihydroxyacetone, erythrulose.

At first glance, it looks like you get much more with the expensive product as opposed to the less expensive one. However, there are some key differences that make one formula the better choice.

## COLORING INGREDIENTS

Both formulas have dihydroxyacetone (DHA). This is critical because it is the ingredient that gives you the brown color. Both formulas also contain caramel, which can potentially have a temporary staining effect. However, the $7 product also contains erythrulose. This ingredient works much like DHA and when mixed together in the same formula it can give a superior color than DHA alone. From a coloring standpoint, the less expensive product is actually better.

## LONGER-LASTING PRODUCT

Another important formula consideration is the thickening system. DHA is a difficult ingredient to work with because it smells bad and can lead to unstable products. The expensive sunless tanner uses sclerotium gum as the thickener. The less expensive formula uses a combination of xanthan gum and aluminum starch octenylsuccinate. The combination in the lower-priced product is actually better.

## OTHER POSSIBLE DIFFERENCES

The other formula differences are ingredients that look good on the label but do not have any real effect when it comes to sunless tanning. Chamomile and aloe look good on a label, but that's about it. If the manufacturers removed those ingredients, you wouldn't notice any difference at all.

## THE BOTTOM LINE

Sunless tanners that actually work all use DHA as the primary ingredient. The price of the product does not reflect how well it works. In fact, the relatively inexpensive sunless tanners found in a drugstore can be superior to more expensive department store brands. Proving once again that when it comes to beauty products, price and performance are not always related.

# IS SEMEN GOOD FOR YOUR SKIN?

**Mandy muses:** *I've heard that semen is good for your skin. Is this true, and if so, why?*

Beauty Brain Sarah Bellum remarked, "What do I think about semen as a skin care ingredient? Well, I don't care much for the product but I love the packaging!" Thanks for the help, Sarah! Now let's get back to the science stuff.

## SEMEN FOR SKIN?

Let's start with an analysis of the components of the substance in question. Semen is composed of seven basic types of chemicals: acids, bases, sugars, enzymes, hormones, proteins and salts.

## ACID TRIP

The acids include organic acids, like citric acid and amino acids. These chemicals have little effect on skin at low levels. The bases include amines, such as putrescine, spermine, spermidine and cadaverine. (Personal note: Putrescine and cadaverine have to be the *least* romantic-sounding chemicals ever!) These bases need to be alkaline to make sure they help the little swimmers get where they need to go. But alkaline doesn't do much for skin. That's the opposite effect you get from alpha hydroxy acids.

## SUGAR AND SPICE

The primary sugar in semen is fructose, which is the main energy source for sperm cells. And while sugar is a good energy source when metabolized by cells, it won't do much when sitting on the surface of your face. At best, it could provide some humectant properties to bind moisture to your skin; at worst, it leaves a sticky film.

Prostaglandin hormones are helpful in procreation because they suppress immune responses caused by foreign bodies—in this case, semen. But there's little benefit associated with applying these hormones topically.

Other components of semen include mucus and texturizing proteins that could conceivably (get it?) form a film on the skin that acts as a moisture reservoir. But, to have a substantial effect, they would have to be spread in a uniform layer across your entire face. (Ewwwwwww!)

## THE BOTTOM LINE

From a skin science point of view, there isn't anything *wrong* with putting semen on your face. It might even provide some minor moisturizing benefit. But there's also no definite advantages (despite what your partner may tell you). A good facial cream (the store-bought kind) will do a much better job with much less social stigma.

# CAN SALIVA CURE ACNE?

**Karina's question:** *My grandmother always told me that putting saliva on my pimples before going to sleep was the best way to get rid of them. Although a lot of people said it was an old wives' tale, it always worked for me. Is there any science to back this up or was I experiencing a placebo effect?*

Karina's grandmother was ahead of her time. A recent report proves what many of us thought all along: There is a specific chemical in human saliva with wound healing properties.

## SALIVA SCIENCE

Scientists originally thought that human saliva contained epidermal growth factor, the same chemical responsible for the healing power of rat saliva. But research from the department of oral biochemistry at the University of Amsterdam has shown that human saliva contains different chemical agents, known as histatins. Using an in vitro model for wound closure, the researchers demonstrated that histatins speed healing.

## COMBATING ACNE

This study focused on wound healing, not pimples. But since acne is caused by a type of bacteria, it is plausible that histatins could be attacking zits at their source. So there is at least a potential scientific explanation for the anti-acne properties of spit. Of course, saliva doesn't magically heal *all* skin injuries.

## THE BOTTOM LINE

Spit on a zit may not be such an old wives' tale after all. Just make sure it's your own saliva!

# DOES THE DERMA ROLLER REALLY WORK?

*Sharon asks:* *What do you think about using a needle-studded product like the derma roller to minimize stretch marks and scars? Supposedly, it stimulates collagen growth and allows products to penetrate more deeply. It sounds pretty risky to me.*

Believe it or not, this kind of needle therapy does have some scientific merit.

## COLLAGEN INDUCTION THERAPY

Poking your skin with a needle-studded roller is technically referred to as percutaneous collagen induction therapy (or CIT). CIT has been used by dermatologists for the last decade or so as a way to reduce wrinkles and scar tissue without significant side effects. Basically, the process involves numbing your face and then poking it with fine needles a few millimeters long. These microperforations spark increased collagen synthesis, which can fill in wrinkles and help heal scars. Other benefits include improved skin tightness, reduced acne scars and stretch marks, as well as fading of scar color.

Amazing, isn't it? Here's how it works: The needles cause an inflammatory response, which triggers a complex series of reactions involving chemotactic factors, neutrophils and fibroblasts. This process leads to the creation of new skin cells that promote collagen deposition. But here's the catch: For this procedure to be effective, the needles need to be at least 1.5 mm long and have a diameter of 0.25 mm. So, because of potential side effects, only a trained dermatologist should administer the procedure.

## DIY DANGER

The distinction in needle length is an important one: Some companies that make these rollers are very clear about the difference between the professional models for medical use and the home models for cosmetic use. But other, less scrupulous companies blur the distinction and imply that the home model will provide all the benefits of the medical treatment. Some are even so bold as to state that their needle rollers will eliminate cellulite and cure baldness.

## THE BOTTOM LINE

Poking your face with needles (when done by a trained professional) is a legitimate way to increase collagen. But the do-it-yourself version is another story altogether. If the roller has the proper type of needles to be effective, then it is a medical device that should only be used by a trained professional. And if it uses smaller needles, then it may be safe for you to use on yourself as an exfoliant, but it won't provide the same collagen-stimulating effect. So, either way, when it comes to DIY face needling, buyer beware!

# THE MAGIC OF WITCH HAZEL

*Jenny just wants to know:* I love a firming skin care product that has witch hazel listed as one of its ingredients. Someone told me that witch hazel is why the product firms but the effects are only temporary, and that, over time, my skin will stop responding to the "firming" action, there will be a rebound effect and my skin will get even looser. Is this true?

Witch hazel is a naturally derived extract made from the bark and leaves of the North American *Hamamelis virginiana* shrub, which grows from Nova Scotia west to Ontario, and south to Texas and Florida. Native Americans used witch hazel for a variety of medicinal purposes. Today it is sold primarily in an alcohol solution under brand names such as Dickinson's. It is widely touted as an astringent.

## WHY USE AN ASTRINGENT?

First, let's talk about what *astringent* really means. Generally speaking, the term is defined as a substance that shrinks or constricts body tissues. For example, the puckery mouth feel you get after drinking red wine is caused by a class of chemicals called tannins. The tannins react with the mucosa in your mouth, causing it to feel tight and rough. In skin care, astringents impart a tightening sensation to the skin.

## HOW DOES WITCH HAZEL WORK ON SKIN?

There are two theories to account for witch hazel's astringent properties. First, it is rich in tannins, which, in theory, can cause a mild coagulation of skin proteins. This coagulation can dry, harden and protect the skin. Second, witch hazel is typically prepared in alcohol, which has a cooling effect on skin due to its low heat of evaporation. This cooling effect can cause a temporary contraction of the skin that feels astringent. Neither of these temporary firming mechanisms has a long-term effect and neither one is likely to produce a "rebound" condition in which your skin will become even looser.

Finally, it's interesting to note that witch hazel is well-studied for its skin protective properties. Many studies have been conducted on this, including one that evaluated witch hazel's ability to treat diaper rash.

## THE BOTTOM LINE

If you've found a skin firming treatment that you like, then stick with it and don't worry about a rebound skin loosening effect. On the other hand, just remember that witch hazel and other astringents won't prevent you from getting serious, long-term wrinkles either.

# WHAT IS SHARK OIL AND WHY IS IT IN SKIN CREAM?

*Jamie's suspicious about squalane: My friend swears by pure squalane oil, but I find it kind of suspicious. Supposedly it's derived from olive oil or shark liver. It's found in quite a few body products, but what exactly does it do?*

To answer your question about squalane, we have to talk about squalene. No, that's not a typo; the e versus the a makes a big difference.

## WHY SHARK LIVER OIL?

Our story begins with squalene, which is a naturally occurring oil that historically has been obtained from sharks' livers. What's so special about shark liver? Sharks belong to a class of fish that do not have a swim bladder to provide buoyancy, so they evolved bodies that contain a lot of lightweight oils to reduce their body's density. That's why their livers are a rich source of squalene.

## SQUALANE VERSUS SQUALENE

Squalene has become a popular ingredient in skin moisturizers because it penetrates the skin quickly, making it feel smooth and soft without leaving a greasy feeling. However, because of its chemical structure, squalene can turn rancid, which is not a good thing in skin cream. So cosmetics formulators, being the crafty chemists that we are, figured out that if we add a couple of hydrogen atoms to the double bonds in squalene we can create a more stable form that still has beneficial properties. This chemically modified version of squalene is called squalane. In today's cosmetics, squalane is much more commonly used than squalene.

## WHERE DOES SQUALANE COME FROM?

Squalane can be made from the squalene that comes from sharks, but there has been pressure from animal rights and environmental groups to find other sources. Today, squalane is produced from a variety of plant sources, including amaranth seed, rice bran, wheat germ and olives.

## THE BOTTOM LINE

While squalene does come from sharks and can improve your skin's condition, the ingredient is not found in cosmetics. Instead, non-shark-derived squalane is used and is moderately effective on skin.

# IS STARCH AN EFFECTIVE SKIN CARE INGREDIENT?

*Rhonda's request:* Can starch work on my skin the same way it does on my clothes; that is, remove the wrinkles?

Anybody who irons clothes knows that starch can help get rid of wrinkles. But what does it do on your skin? Let's begin with a quick review of some of the different types of starches used in cosmetic products.

## STARCHED-BASED COSMETICS

Simple starches that are used in cosmetics are most frequently made from rice, potato, corn or even tapioca. These can be chemically modified to create ingredients such as hydroxypropyl starch phosphate or aluminum starch octenylsuccinate. In powdered products, these starches can impart a smooth, velvety feel and help prevent caking. In creams and lotions they can give the product a creamier, richer texture; reduce greasiness; improve the feel of the product on your skin; and even help stabilize the emulsion so the product has a longer shelf life.

## CAN STARCH ELIMINATE WRINKLES?

Some types of starch are good film formers. When formulated into the right kind of skin cream, they can leave a thin film on your face that provides a tightening effect as it dries. This film can temporarily give the impression of reducing wrinkles, but when you wash your face, the starch goes away and the wrinkles return.

## THE BOTTOM LINE

Starch is a very powerful natural (or at least naturally derived) ingredient that helps make cosmetics work better. And while it may even temporarily help give your skin a tighter texture, starch will not banish wrinkles.

# CAN AVON ANEW GET RID OF CROW'S-FEET?

**Donna asks:** *I've heard that Avon is claiming that their Anew product will reduce or eliminate crow's feet. This sounds too good to be true. Is it?*

Avon Anew Clinical Crow's Feet Corrector is a good illustration of the power of cosmetic marketing and advertising. You might get the impression that Avon claims the product can "reduce or eliminate crow's-feet," but upon further investigation, that's not exactly what the packaging says. To figure out whether this product really works, you need to look at Avon's claims.

## AVON ANEW CLINICAL'S CLAIMS

On their website, here's what Avon says about their Anew Clinical Crow's Feet Corrector:

1. The first 2-in-1 treatment to resurface & visibly fill crow's feet…at home.

2. Professional crow's feet laser treatments can be painful and costly (up to $2000 per treatment).

3. Anew Clinical Crow's Feet Corrector is a specialized eye treatment system uniquely formulated to smooth out and fill in lines around the delicate eye area — no doctors, no lasers.

4. *In just three days\** crow's feet lines look plumped out and leveled.

5. *Over time 100 percent\*\** of women showed a reduction in the length, depth and number of crow's feet wrinkles.

The last two statements make numerical claims that require specific support. The asterisks indicate that a consumer panel was used to support the claim that crow's-feet "look" plumped out and leveled. This is a common testing method in the cosmetics industry. Unfortunately, we think it's biased in favor of the cosmetics companies, and usually ends up substantiating the claims they want to make. Most study participants will naturally rate any product as effective. They want to solve the problem and will take any change, no matter how small, as an indication of improvement in their condition. As long as the product isn't tested against a placebo control, it's simple to get high ratings.

The claim that 100 percent of women showed a reduction in crow's-feet is supported by a dermatologist-supervised clinical evaluation. These studies are designed and conducted in a clinical setting under a doctor's supervision. The dermatologist either personally rates the number and intensity of the panelists' wrinkles, or the rating is conducted by a technician and the dermatologist reviews the results before they are published. The best studies are done as randomized, double-blinded clinical trials where neither the panelists nor the researchers know who was treated with the control or the test product. This methodology ensures the results are honest because no one knows the "right" answer.

## CROW'S-FEET CREDIBILITY

The ability of a product to impact the appearance of fine lines and wrinkles is nothing new. This can be achieved through a combination of plumping up the skin with moisturizing agents and tightening the skin with film form agents. What makes Anew Clinical's claim seem so impressive is that Avon is implying their results are comparable to those you'd achieve from a doctor-administered laser treatment. Such treatments not only resurface the top layers of skin but can also stimulate collagen production at deeper levels.

## THE BOTTOM LINE

It's very plausible that Avon Anew can reduce the appearance of fine lines and wrinkles around the eye area. It's ridiculous for them to expect us to think it can replace surgical procedures.

# CAN MESOTHERAPY MELT AWAY FAT?

**Deb asks:** *What do you know about a procedure for skin tightening known as mesotherapy? Apparently, it has been used for many years in France and recently came to the United States. It is a series of injections with a drug "cocktail" containing homeopathic treatments and chemicals (including hyaluronic acid) to stimulate skin tightening and collagen production.*

According to the American Society of Plastic Surgeons (via *Science Daily*), mesotherapy has not been established as safe and effective: "There is no information on what happens to fatty acids once they leave the targeted area or how the various ingredients affect the body's organs and other tissues. There is simply too much we do not know about mesotherapy to say it is unquestionably safe for patients."

Similarly, in a 2008 paper published in the journal *Aesthetic Plastic Surgery*, the authors opined that even though mesotherapy is growing in popularity, the results it provides and the risks it presents are at best "ambiguous." They registered their concern that independent medical professionals who have reviewed the data are skeptical due to both the lack of confirmed efficacy and the potential for side effects.

## THE BOTTOM LINE

Considering the lack of solid medical data on this process, we'd be very careful. There isn't enough evidence to say conclusively that mesotherapy is worth doing.

# IS IT SAFE TO USE LIPSTICK ON YOUR CHEEKS?

*Stephanie wants to know:* Is it safe to use makeup for other things than origi-nally intended? I know some people use lipstick on their cheeks, but what about eye shadow? Can you use it (in red shades, of course) as lipstick or blush? Can you use lipstick on your eyes? Lip liner as eyeliner and vice versa?

We can't think of any significant danger posed by using eye makeup or lipstick on your face. The only thing that *might* be a problem is using products on your lips that weren't meant to be used there. That's because lipsticks and lip glosses are made with ingredients that are meant for incidental ingestion (that means it's OK to swallow small amounts). The same is not true for eye or face makeup. But the real potential danger is in using lip and face stuff on your eyes!

## LIP LINER AS EYELINER?

This is a no-no! There are some ingredients that are used in face makeup that are not permitted to be used in eye makeup for safety reasons. The two most com-mon examples are colors and preservatives. There are only a few colorants that are approved for use around the eyes, while products for the lips and the face can in-corporate many, many more. The other thing to consider is bacterial contamination. While some bacteria in your lip gloss won't kill you if you ingest it, the same bacteria in your eye could cause infection or even blindness! This is an even greater danger if you're using a product like a mascara wand that can scratch the surface of your eye. So stick to eye products and be safe!

## THE BOTTOM LINE

While cosmetics in general are very safe, you do need to be extra cautious when applying products to your eyes.

# DO DRYER SHEETS CAUSE ACNE?

**Nina asks:** *Is it true that dryer sheets can cause acne? I've also heard they contain known carcinogens and are toxic. If so, can enough of the toxic chemicals make their way onto our skin from clothing, towels and other laundry and cause harm? I smell some scare tactics.*

One must be careful when declaring that a chemical is "toxic." Many substances can be toxic (or carcinogenic) under certain use conditions (e.g., when ingesting or inhaling high concentrations over long periods). But that doesn't necessarily mean that indirect contact with a small amount is problematic.

## FABRIC SOFTENER SICKNESS?

Checking the literature for specific research on the health effects of dryer sheets, we found that testing done on Bounce brand dryer sheets showed that they "produced no irritation in challenge patch tests, provocative patch tests, continuous patch tests, repeated insult patch tests, prick tests and clinical wear tests. Bounce would not be expected to cause irritation or induce cutaneous sensitization." However, we did find one PubMed study showing that people with chemical sensitivity did have some reaction when exposed to dryer sheet chemicals, compared to a control group of chemicals. That's not much information to go on, but without more research, we would have to say that it is safe for most people to use Bounce and that it would be prudent to avoid using fabric softeners if you are sensitive to chemicals and have a high level of concern.

## BREAKOUTS FROM BOUNCE?

To determine if dryer sheets cause acne there are two key questions that must be answered: (1) Are the chemicals used on dryer sheets comedogenic (that is, do they cause acne?); and (2) are those chemicals transferred to the skin in sufficient quantities to have any effect?

First, what chemicals are used in dryer sheets? It's impossible to say for any given product because household products, unlike cosmetics, don't have to provide a list of ingredients. But two common types of dryer sheet ingredients are softening agents (like dihydrogenated tallow dimethyl ammonium chloride and polydimethylsiloxane) as well as waxy coating agents (like stearic acid). Siloxanes (or silicones in general) and stearic acid rate very low on the comedogenicity scale. So these specific ingredients would be highly unlikely to cause breakouts. But without a

# THE TOP 10 INGREDIENTS THAT IRRITATE THE SKIN

Temporary skin rash, reddening or itchiness is known as allergic contact dermatitis, and a study by the Mayo Clinic cites the top ten ingredients that can cause the condition. The list includes metals, antibiotics, fragrance ingredients and various preservatives. The study was done using a method called patch testing, in which human volunteers allow researchers to stick patches of these chemicals on their bodies for hours and days on end.

If you experience this condition, check the ingredients list on your beauty and skin care products and avoid those that contain any of the following:

1. **Nickel** (nickel sulfate hexahydrate): Found in jewelry or on your clothes.

2. **Gold** (gold sodium thiosulfate): Yes, the same stuff used to make jewelry.

3. **Cobalt chloride:** A metal used in many applications, like medical products, hair dye and antiperspirants, to name a few.

4. **Neomycin sulfate:** An antibiotic used in various first aid creams. Less commonly used in cosmetics.

5. **Bacitracin:** Another antibiotic.

6. **Thimerosal:** A preservative ingredient used in antiseptics and vaccines.

7. **Balsam of Peru** (myroxylon pereirae): A natural fragrance ingredient derived from tree resin, and used in perfumes and skin lotions. Who said "natural" was better?

8. **Fragrance mix:** Common fragrance allergens found in cosmetic products. Manufacturers in the United States must list this on the ingredients statement.

9. **Formaldehyde:** A much-maligned preservative. You might remember the smell of this stuff from high school biology class.

10. **Quaternium-15:** Another preservative used in some cosmetics.

complete list of ingredients, it's impossible to know the true acne-genic potential of any given dryer sheet formulation.

Second, how much of these ingredients actually end up on your skin? Let's assume we're talking about drying your face with a towel that you dried with a fabric softener sheet. The small amount of softening formula on a dryer sheet is spread across an entire dryer load of towels. And using one of those towels to dry your face will only transfer to your face a tiny fraction of the total material on the towel. So the amount of chemicals deposited on your skin is very low. Even for those chemicals that do cause acne, a very low dose is unlikely to clog pores. While there haven't been any published studies on this topic, our guess is that the likelihood of dryer sheets causing acne is very, very slight.

## THE BOTTOM LINE

While there are no definitive answers to these questions, there doesn't seem to be a need for a high level of concern. If you're still not convinced, just stop using dryer sheets. Most clothes and towels are soft enough without them.

# THE SURPRISING SECRET OF SOAP

*Maggie asks:* Is a bar of soap a cosmetic or a drug? And what about soap in liquid form?

See page 156 about the difference between cosmetics and drugs. While the Food, Drug and Cosmetic Act classifies other personal cleansing products as either cosmetics or drugs, soap is neither. Why?

## SOAPY SECRET

Even though the FD&C Act defines "articles for cleansing" as cosmetics, soap is technically exempt from that law. The reason is political: At the time the original law was passed (1906), soap manufacturers successfully lobbied to be excluded from the definition of "cosmetic" just as ice cream companies wanted to be excluded from labeling requirements for foods. So, in the government's eyes, soap is neither a cosmetic *nor* a drug. Instead, it's given its own definition.

## DEFINITION OF SOAP

To be soap, a product must meet two criteria:

1.  It must be primarily made from the alkali salt of fatty acids.

2.  It must be labeled, sold and represented solely as soap.

If a cleansing product does not meet these criteria, then it is not really soap—it's either a drug or a cosmetic. Think of it this way: You could have different cleansing bars that all look and act like a bar of soap, but they could be classified differently depending on what ingredients they contain and what claims they make. If the first bar is made of synthetic detergents instead of fatty acids, it may be called a soap, but it is regulated as a cosmetic. (Cosmetics must have ingredients lists; soaps do not.) If the second bar makes claims about moisturizing skin, then it is a cosmetic. And if the third bar contains an active drug and/or makes claims about treating skin conditions (like acne), then it is a drug. Get it?

## WHAT ABOUT LIQUID SOAPS?

Liquid soaps are not really soaps at all! Because they are not made with neutralized fatty acids, they are actually cosmetics and are regulated under the FD&C Act, even though they may have the word *soap* in their name.

## THE BOTTOM LINE

Politics and science make strange bedfellows, which is why soaps can be either drugs or cosmetics. Or they can be just...soap!

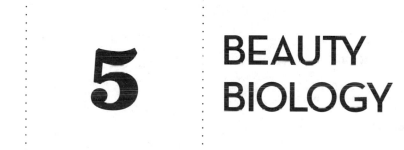

# 5 BEAUTY BIOLOGY

To figure out if a cure for any skin problem could work, it's important to know what is causing the problem in the first place. In this chapter we explore the causes of wrinkles, acne, enlarged pores, darkened skin and rosacea. You'll learn the proper way to pop a pimple, how to reduce enlarged pores and even how to eliminate darkened armpits.

# FOUR TYPES OF WRINKLES AND HOW TO GET RID OF THEM

*Irene inquires:* *Cosmetics companies don't usually do a good job of explaining the problems they claim to solve. Take antiwrinkle creams, for example. Can some-one please tell me what causes wrinkles in the first place?*

Researchers at the University Hospital of Liege, Belgium determined that there are actually four distinctly different types of wrinkles that you'll (eventually) have to face.

## 1. ATROPHIC CRINKLING RHYTIDS

*What are they?*
Fine lines on the face that are almost parallel to each other.

*Where do they occur?*
They show up in different areas of the face and body, but they tend to disappear when skin is stretched transversally (that means they shift when your body posture changes). These wrinkles are associated with a loss of elasticity.

*What can you do?*
Since these wrinkles are due to an underlying loss of collagen, you need to protect your skin by using sun protectants. You can also use moisturizers to temporarily plump the skin and diminish the appearance of these fine lines.

## 2. PERMANENT ELASTIC CREASES

*What are they?*
These are crease lines in the skin that become increasingly permanent over time, especially with sun exposure.

*Where do they occur?*
They show up most frequently on the cheek, the upper lip and the base of the neck.

*What can you do?*
Sun exposure makes this type of wrinkle worse. So unless you're blessed with natu-rally dark skin, you should avoid sun exposure or use a sunscreen on these areas to prevent this kind of wrinkling.

## 3. DYNAMIC EXPRESSION LINES

*What are they?*

Wrinkles that are caused by facial muscle movement.

*Where do they occur?*

On the forehead (frown lines) and around the eyes (crow's-feet).

*What can you do?*

These wrinkles respond to Botox or similar treatments.

## 4. GRAVITATIONAL FOLDS

*What are they?*

As the name implies, these lines stem from the effects of gravity, and they become increasingly obvious as skin begins to fold and sag.

*Where do they occur?*

The location of these wrinkles is related to the thickness of a person's skin. While we would have thought this means that thicker skin shows more folds, surprisingly research shows that a fat face may have fewer gravity folds than a lean face.

*What can you do?*

Facelifting procedures are effective at removing these kinds of wrinkles.

Unfortunately, wrinkles are a reality of life. Gravity, natural UV radiation and genetics all conspire against us to create them. There is only so much you can do with cosmetics to remove them, which is why so many people turn to surgery when they are really desperate. Perhaps the best thing you can do is learn to accept how your body looks. At least until scientists can come up with better solutions.

# WHAT CAUSES ACNE AND CAN SKINTACTIX CURE IT?

*Lydia longs to learn:* Skintactix claims to have a very interesting combination of cleansers in its acne treatment products, and its website talks very scientifically about how each works not only to kill the bacteria causing acne, but also to stop the process of inflammation at a molecular level. As someone who has struggled with acne since I was a teen, that thought intrigued me. Do you think that these ingredients can really stop inflammation and, if so, why don't dermatologists use it?

## TYPES OF ACNE

First, you have to realize that there are two kinds of acne: noninflammatory and inflammatory. Second, you have to realize that for acne to occur, three conditions must be met:

**1** **Oil glands gone wild**
Your sebaceous glands begin to produce an excessive amount of oil. This increase in oil production is typically, but not always, associated with a change in hormones. That's why teenagers get so many zits, but it can strike adults as well. Either way, the result is that the ducts in your dermis are filled with more oily sebum than usual.

**2** **Chunky skin is gunky**
Your skin cells don't shed properly. Normally your dead skin cells, which are made of keratin, flake off in very tiny pieces that don't cause any problems. But sometimes they go haywire and start to grow so quickly that they don't flake off properly. When that happens, those chunks of cells can mechanically block the outward flow of sebum.

**3** **Bad bacterial blockage**
This is caused by the organism *Propionibacterium* acnes (aka *P.* acnes), which thrives in the lipid-rich sebum in your oil glands. These bacteria feed off the oil and grow and grow and grow…

When the first two conditions are met, the excess sebum and the dead keratin cells clog your oil duct by forming a follicular plug called a microcomedo. (That's where the term *comedogenic* comes from, get it?) This tiny plug is the first sign of acne. As more and more gunk fills up the duct, the walls of the hair follicle become swollen and distended.

What was a microcomedo now becomes a larger comedo, also known as a whitehead. As the plug continues to grow, it starts to poke through the opening of the oil duct and becomes visible as a blackhead. (Blackheads look black because they contain melanin, the same pigment in your skin that's responsible for your suntan.) Whiteheads and blackheads are technically known as noninflammatory acne.

In inflammatory acne, the comedo becomes inflamed and turns into a raised, reddened pus-engorged bump. What, you ask, makes the noninflammatory type turn inflammatory? The culprit is lipase, a chemical produced by excessive growth of the *P. acnes* bacteria. The lipase breaks down the oily triglycerides in your skin, releasing fatty acids. These acids irritate the skin and cause inflammation. (That process has to do with the release of hydrolytic enzymes that break down the follicular wall. But we'll save that story for another time.) Suffice it to say that these acids can turn a simple blackhead into an oozing, pus-filled volcano.

## WHAT'S IN SKINTACTIX?
This Skintactix line consists primarily of surfactant-based cleansers and exfoliants that use salicylic acid as their active ingredient. They also contain several plant extracts, like cinnamon, sage and thyme. The Skintactix website is not exactly clear about the precise purpose of these ingredients, but the implication is that they are anti-inflammatory agents.

## DO SKINTACTIX PRODUCTS WORK?
Well, sal acid is an approved anti-acne agent, so we'd expect these products would work as well as similar products on the market. But we can't find any clinical data that suggest the plant extracts they contain have been proven effective against acne inflammation.

## ANTI-INFLAMMATORY ACNE FIGHTERS
You asked why dermatologists don't use anti-inflammatory agents. Well, in reality, they do. The most popularly prescribed anti-acne antibiotics (Tetracycline, Meclocycline, Erythromycin, Clindamycin, Tretinoin) do have anti-inflammatory properties. So when your doctor prescribes this kind of medicine for your zits, you're really getting a two-for-one effect: antibiotic and anti-inflammatory. If you have a ton of inflamed blackheads, the Beauty Brains think you may need to see your doctor for a prescription.

## THE BOTTOM LINE

While the salicylic acid in Skintactix will be effective for treating acne, there is no evidence that the plant extracts in their formulas will have any added benefits.

# HOW TO POP A PIMPLE

*Margie's worried:* I have always been told that it's unhealthy and potentially damaging to squeeze my own zits. I can't afford to hire people to squeeze my pimples on a regular basis. Am I really damaging my skin forever if I pop a pimple? Am I any less qualified to pick at my zits than an esthetician? It doesn't seem like rocket science to me.

By squeezing your own zits you might, indeed, make them worse. According to the American Academy of Dermatologists, you should *not* pick, scratch, pop or squeeze pimples yourself because you'll get more redness, swelling, inflammation and possible scarring. (If you want to learn more about the causes and effects of acne, see page 92).

But, if you *insist* on throwing caution to the wind and picking those pus pockets yourself, here are some tips:

**Seven easy steps to popping your own pimples (courtesy of acne.org)**

1. Take a warm shower or bath to soften your skin.
2. Wash your face and remove all makeup.
3. Wash your hands to prevent spreading germs and infecting the pimple.
4. Sterilize a needle (a dirty needle will cause an infection and maybe a bigger pimple).
5. Gently prick the tip of the pimple with the needle.
6. Take a clean tissue or piece of toilet paper and wrap it around your index fingers.
7. Gently apply pressure to the sides of the pimple to ease out the pus. Stop when blood or clear fluid comes out.

# THE RED-FACED REGRET OF ROSACEA

*Victoria has cause for concern:* I have clusters of dry, red, raised bumps on both sides of my chin. I've been using hydrocortisone, which helps, but doesn't cure the problem. I also have a flush to my cheeks and am prone to blushing, which are two characteristics of rosacea. Does this sound like rosacea and do you know of any better remedies than hydrocortisone?

## WHAT IS ROSACEA?

Rosacea is an inflammatory skin condition that causes the skin around your nose, cheeks, chin and eyes to become very red and flushed. Over 14 million Americans suffer from this neurovascular disorder, according to the National Rosacea Society. Why is this disorder disturbing? Because it's more than just a simple case of being red-faced! The condition has psychological effects as well. The society has done studies that show that nearly 70 percent of rosacea sufferers have low self-esteem, and 41 percent say that the condition causes them to avoid public contact or cancel social engagements.

## WHAT CAUSES ROSACEA?

No one knows for sure what causes rosacea, but there are several theories. It could be related to how facial blood vessels cope with being flushed and dilated. Or it could be that it's an overactive inflammatory response to some unknown pathogen. Though the exact cause is unknown, we do know that it can be worsened by harsh skin treatments, strong acne medications and even exposure to excessive sunlight.

## HOW CAN YOU TELL IF YOU HAVE ROSACEA?

You should consult your dermatologist to find out if your condition really is rosacea, but here are some common symptoms you can look for. The redness associated with rosacea primarily occurs in the flushing zone—the nose, cheeks, chin and forehead. Besides the reddening, you may see dilated blood vessels and facial swelling. You may also feel a slight burning sensation on your face. Inflammatory papules and pustules (the red bumps) may develop as well.

You should also note that rosacea starts as mild episodes of facial blushing or flushing, which can turn into a permanently red face over time.

There is a special type of rosacea, known as ocular rosacea, that affects both the eye surface and the eyelid. This condition can cause redness, dry eyes, crusting and even loss of eyelashes.

## WHAT CAN YOU DO ABOUT ROSACEA?

We didn't find any reference to using hydrocortisone to fight rosacea, but there are other medications that are used to control the redness and reduce the number of papules and pustules.

The most commonly used drugs are oral antibiotics and topical metronidazole. Isotretinoin (Accutane) has also been shown to work against severe papopustular rosacea because it physically shrinks sebaceous glands and it has potent anti-inflammatory properties. And there has been some discussion that topical application of a drug called Finacea may be a promising treatment as well. You'll need a prescription from your doctor for all of these, though.

There are some things you can do without a prescription: According to the experts, you should use a gentle cleansing regimen to avoid aggravating the condition. So make sure you're using a mild facial cleanser and not scrubbing too much! You should also limit sun exposure by protecting your skin with a good nonirritating sunscreen every day. You might find that a product that contains physical sunblock ingredients like zinc oxide or titanium dioxide might be less aggravating than some of the reactive sunscreens.

For much, much more on this subject, visit the Rosacea Support Group at www.rosacea-support.org.

# WHAT'S THE DIFFERENCE BETWEEN ANTIPERSPIRANT AND DEODORANT?

*Patty's perspiration puzzle:* What's the difference between antiperspirant and deodorant and which should I be using?

Antiperspirants, as the name implies, stop you from perspiring, or sweating. Deodorants simply get rid of odor. Ultimately, both products are trying to do the same thing: stop you from being stinky. But the way they carry out their deodorizing duty differs.

### WHY DOES SWEAT SMELL BAD?

Before we explain how these products work, let's talk a little bit about perspiration. It works like this: You sweat and bacteria grow in the moist, warm areas where the sweat collects. When the bacteria grow, they eat some of the stuff in your sweat (primarily fatty acids) and they poop out stuff that smells bad. End result? BO.

## WHAT DO DEODORANTS DO?

Deodorants contain an active ingredient (triclosan is the most commonly used one) that prevents the bacteria from growing and devouring your sweat. No bacteria = no body odor. However, you still get wet pits.

## HOW DO ANTIPERSPIRANTS ACT?

Antiperspirants, on the other hand, fight the odor problem in a different way. The active ingredients in antiperspirants, typically zinc salts, interact with your sweat glands to stop perspiration. No perspiration = no food for bacteria = no body odor.

## IS IT BAD TO PLUG YOUR PORES?

OK, we know what you're thinking: Isn't it bad for you to plug your sweat glands like that? Don't sweat it. But seriously, it's not something you need to worry about. You're only affecting a small portion of your body's sweat glands, so you're not interfering with your body's natural cooling mechanism.

Antiperspirants also have some mild antibacterial properties, so if you do still sweat a little bit, not much bacteria will grow. And, by the way, both antiperspirants and deodorants also contain fragrance to cover up any odor that does sneak through.

## WET OR DRY—HOW DO YOU DECIDE?

So there you have it—two different approaches to solving the same problem. Which one should you use? That's really up to you. Are your armpits sensitive as a result of shaving? You might want to use a deodorant because some antiperspirants can irritate freshly shaved skin. Do you really, really, really sweat a lot? Then you might need an antiperspirant to avoid dripping. Do you wear black dresses that get white stains from antiperspirants? A clear deodorant might be the way to go.

## THE BOTTOM LINE

The difference between antiperspirant and deodorant is all about sweating. Antiperspirant stops it, while deodorant doesn't. Both of them fight body odor.

# WHY ARMPIT HAIR DOESN'T GROW DOWN TO YOUR KNEES

*Laura longs to learn: How does hair know when to grow? When you shave your legs, it grows back, but it stops growing after a certain length. If you shave it again, it will grow back to that length. What's up with that?*

The first thing to understand is that hair goes through three different stages as it grows: anagen, catagen and telogen phases. The anagen stage (that's anagen, not Anakin!) is the stage where the hair grows like crazy. This stage can last four to six years and can produce scalp hairs that grow to be almost three feet in length! And if you think three feet is impressive, you ain't seen nothin'! Human scalp hair longer than five feet has been reported! Yikes! We'd hate to see the bill from *her* stylist!

The catagen stage follows the anagen stage. This is basically a transitional stage, which means the follicle is slowing down production of the hair—not much happens here.

The third stage is the telogen, or resting, stage. The hair stops growing and just sits there in the follicle. When the cycle starts all over again with the anagen phase, the old hair is pushed out by the new hair. That's one of the reasons you normally shed about 100 or so hairs each day—the old ones are getting replaced by the new ones.

## TYPES OF HAIRS

The second thing to understand is that there are two different types of hairs: terminal and vellus. Terminal are long hairs (the three-footers we mentioned), which are thicker and have a longer growing cycle of six to eight years, meaning most of the time they are in the anagen phase. Terminal hairs are the kind you have to cut because they get too long and are mostly found on the scalp.

Vellus, on the other hand, are short hairs (a millimeter or less) that are very fine, and have a very short life cycle, which means they spend most of the time in the telogen phase. That also means they'll never grow as long as scalp hair. These very fine hairs are found on "hairless" parts of the body like arms and legs. (OK, those areas aren't hairless, but they kind of look hairless because the hairs are so tiny and fine.)

## THE BOTTOM LINE

Hair growth is determined by the type of hair and the stage of growth it's in. Which, of course, is determined by hormones. Isn't everything?

# WHAT'S THE DIFFERENCE BETWEEN SKIN IRRITATION AND SKIN ALLERGIES?

*Gloria is grumbling:* I have severe allergies to dust and pollen and it really bugs me when I hear my friends say they're "allergic" to cosmetics. I don't think they're allergic—I think the cosmetics are probably just irritating their skin. Please tell me who's right.

Actually you *and* your friends might both be right. Certain chemicals in cosmetics can cause negative reactions in some people. There are two basic types of reactions: irritation reaction (also known as irritant contact dermatitis, or ICD) and allergic response (also known as allergic contact dermatitis, or ACD). In general terms, irritation occurs when your cells are attacked by harsh chemicals. An allergy occurs when your immune system develops antibodies in response to a chemical you've been exposed to (as in hay fever).

It's important to understand if you're irritated or allergic because it will help your doctor determine the right course of treatment. Here's how you can tell the difference.

## WHAT THEY DO TO YOUR SKIN

Irritation Gives you redness with possible oozing sores. Your skin may develop a chapped, glazed or scaled appearance. You'll feel burning, stinging, pain and soreness. You may also have some itchiness.

Allergies The skin appearance may be similar to irritation, but the main symptom is itchiness.

## WHERE THE RESPONSE OCCURS

Irritation The effects are usually limited to the part of the skin that came in contact with the chemical.

Allergies Because you're producing antibodies, the effects are not limited to the contact point. The effects may be worse in the contact area, but you can develop symptoms anywhere on your body.

## HOW LONG IT TAKES FOR THE RESPONSE TO DEVELOP

Irritation Symptoms develop after a single exposure. They usually appear in a few minutes—or at most within a few hours—after contact.

<u>Allergies</u> After the first exposure, you typically have no symptoms. That's because your body hasn't developed an antibody response to the agent yet. After subsequent exposures, symptoms may take 24 to 72 hours to develop.

# 5 WAYS TO REDUCE ENLARGED PORES

At first glance, you may think that pore control products offer to make your pores smaller, but if you read the label carefully, you'll see that in most cases they just claim to reduce the appearance of large pores. That may sound like a subtle distinction, but it's not. There's not much you can do to physically make your pores smaller, but you can avoid making them look larger. Instead of looking for "shrinking" products, try avoiding these factors that can make pores look plump:

1. **Skin debris** like dead skin cells can collect in pores, making them appear bigger. Good facial cleansing is the key to staying debris-free.

2. **Excessive oiliness** can keep pores filled with a layer of oil that accentuates their appearance. Consider using oil-absorbing makeup or doing more frequent cleansing or blotting.

3. **Bacterial growth** contributes to blackheads and makes pores appear freakishly huge. Exfoliation can help.

4. **Sun exposure** can thicken the skin cells around the edge of pores, making them appear larger. Using a sunscreen or limiting your sun exposure is a good idea.

5. **Genetics** determines your skin type and if you're unlucky enough to be born with oily, thicker skin, your pores will probably be more noticeable. Unfortunately, there is not much you can do about this.

## THE BOTTOM LINE

People can be both allergic to and irritated by chemicals in cosmetics. It's usually assumed that they are the same thing, but there are differences, and only a doctor can tell for sure.

# TOP FIVE CAUSES OF DARKENED ARMPITS

*Germaine is puzzled by her pits:* What causes darkened armpits and what can I do to get rid of them? They're so embarrassing!

It's not surprising that so many people have this problem—there are at least five different reasons your pits may be darker than they should be.

**1 Shaving**
When you shave, you cut the hairs off at, or just below, the surface of the skin. If your hairs are slightly darker than your skin color, it can appear as though your skin has a dark stain when it's really just subsurface hair.

*What to do about it:* Stop shaving and try waxing or plucking instead, so you get rid of the hair below the skin surface. Since the hairs aren't lurking so close to the top of your skin, they won't be as visible.

**2 Buildup of dead skin cells**
According to at least one dermatologist, dark spots under your arms are the result of dead skin cells that are trapped in microscopic "hills and valleys" on your skin.

*What to do about it:* Exfoliate, preferably with a product containing lactic acid.

**3 Antiperspirant and deodorant usage**
In theory, some ingredients in these products (perhaps the fragrance) could be reacting with the skin to cause discoloration. Practically speaking, this seems unlikely, but many people do claim that when they stop using these products, the darkness goes away.

*What to do about it:* Try switching brands or using a deodorant instead of an antiperspirant.

**4** **A medical condition called acanthosis nigricans**
This condition causes light-brown-to-black markings on the neck, under the arms or in the groin. It can be related to insulin production or to a glandular disorder, and it typically occurs in people who are overweight.

*What to do about it:* Watch your diet in order to control insulin production and see your doctor about using Retin-A, 20% urea, alpha hydroxy acids or salicylic acid prescriptions to lighten your armpits.

**5** **Hyperpigmentation**
This condition causes your skin to produce excess melanin pigment. It doesn't usually affect armpits, so it's a less likely cause.

*What to do about it:* Use a skin bleaching cream to destroy the excess melanin. We don't recommend this unless you consult a dermatologist first. You can also try laser treatment to destroy the pigment.

# PART III

# MAKEUP

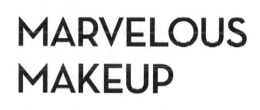

# 6 MARVELOUS MAKEUP

Is your blush really interacting with your skin's DNA or is it chemical trickery produced by clever beauty marketers? In this chapter we answer questions about the mysteries of makeup.

# CAN YOU GET HOOKED ON LIP BALM?

**Chris is curious:** *Is it really possible to be addicted to lip balm?*

Lip balm users have been wondering about this for generations. It's such a popular topic that there's even a website, www.lipbalmanonymous.com, devoted to finding the answer!

The conversation makes for entertaining reading, but the one argument that we did *not* see discussed is, in our opinion, the most scientifically valid one. It goes something like this.

## SKIN SIGNALS FOR NEW CELLS

Skin is a very complicated organ with multiple layers. The top layer, the stratum corneum, consists mainly of dead, dried-up cells. As those cells die and flake off, they send a signal to a deeper layer of skin (called the basal layer) to produce fresh skin cells. This is a very simplified description of the process called cellular turnover. (Contrary to what you might have thought, "cellular turnover" does *not* refer to switching your mobile phone plan.)

## LIP BALM SLOWS DOWN THE SIGNAL

When you apply lip balm, you're creating a barrier layer that prevents, or at least retards, the evaporation of moisture from the inner layers of skin. Since the top layer isn't drying and flaking off as much, the basal layer never gets the signal to produce new cells.

## YOUR SKIN HAS TO CATCH UP

But when you stop using the lip balm, all of a sudden your lips dry out and your basal layer has to hurry up and start producing new cells. But since your lips already feel dry again, you add more lip balm, which once again tells the basal layer, "Hey, everything's fine up here on the surface—we don't need any more new skin cells."

## THE CYCLE REPEATS

But, of course, once that application of lip balm has worn off and there are no new, plump, moist skin cells to replace the ones that are drying out, your lips feel dry again and you have to add more lip balm. And so on, and so on…Get the picture? That's why you feel addicted to lip balm—you've "trained" your body to rely on it!

## THE BOTTOM LINE

It's not an addiction in the true medical sense, but, yes, you can train your body to rely on lip balm. Then you'll have trouble giving it up.

# DO EYE CREAMS REALLY REDUCE CIRCLES AND PUFFINESS?

*Lucy longingly asks:* I just bought Eyecon from Benefit, but I'm not sure if it's really doing anything. What are eye creams and is their claim of reducing under-eye circles and puffiness at all valid? What ingredients should I look for in an eye cream for these things?

Do eye creams really do what they say they'll do? Well, the answer is a little bit yes, a little bit no. All skin creams (should) moisturize. But eye creams have some added responsibilities.

**1** **Moisturization**
They've got to moisturize without adding a lot of heaviness or greasiness. After all, it's likely that you'll apply some kind of makeup around your eyes and you don't want an eye cream to interfere with your foundation, for example.

**2** **Mildness**
They need to be extra mild, since the area around the eye is particularly sensitive to irritation. Fragrance-free is best.

**3** **Tightening**
They should tighten the skin around the eyes, since they claim to reduce wrinkles. While they can't work miracles, they can do this to some extent by adding polymers that form a film on the skin as they dry. This film can make the skin look and feel a little bit tighter.

The Eyecon product you cited seems designed to do just that. It contains ingredients like ethylene/acrylic acid copolymer, butylene glycol, glyceryl polymethacrylate and sodium polyacrylate. These are all film-forming agents that can help eyes feel less puffy and look less wrinkled.

Of course, the effect varies from person to person; even in best-case scenarios it may not be dramatically noticeable; and even if it does work it's only a temporary fix at best. But if you notice enough difference, you might want to continue using the product.

Want another opinion? Paula Begoun, the Cosmetic Cop, has a much harsher opinion of eye creams. She says that they are no different from facial moisturizers and that they are "a whim of the cosmetics industry designed to evoke the sale of two products when only one is needed."

## THE BOTTOM LINE

Eye creams are essentially moisturizers that are modified for use on the thin skin around the eyes. While they don't work miracles, as they claim, they do contain ingredients that may offer some temporary benefit. We say try them and see what you think. But as always, buyer beware.

# DO LIP PLUMPERS REALLY WORK?

*Jessie just wants to know: I recently tried a lip plumper while browsing in Sephora. I was skeptical, but then as I walked around the store, I really did notice my lips feeling slightly fuller and very tingly. Was this my imagination? What are lip plumpers and how do they work?*

Lip plumpers work by temporarily irritating lips and causing them to swell slightly. That tingly feeling is not your imagination; it's your lips reacting to a menthol-type chemical that most plumpers use. The effect is slight and temporary—don't expect to look like you've had a collagen injection.

And while these products do have this effect, the bad news is that it's not really good for your lips to use them on a regular basis because they can be damaging to the skin. Look for menthoxypropanediol on the ingredients list if you're not sure the product will really plump or not.

## THE BOTTOM LINE

Lip plumpers will temporarily make your lips look more full. But don't expect miracles and don't use them too often as they can be damaging.

# IS YOUR LIP PLUMPER MAKING YOU SICK?

*Mildred is miserable:* Recently, I had a terrible allergic reaction on my lips to the Primal Elements Lip Plumper. Shortly after putting it on, I had severe swelling, bumps and peeling. My dermatologist prescribed cortisone cream, which seems to be working but it will be a while until it's completely healed. What could have caused this reaction? Maybe the cinnamon?

We looked at the ingredients list of this product and have some theories about which ingredients might be the problem.

## SPICY HOT?

Cinnamon is a good guess because cinnamic aldehyde, a component of cinnamon oil, is known to cause allergic contact dermatitis. Symptoms include a rash, intense swelling and redness of the affected area.

However, that doesn't seem to be the likely culprit for your lip plumper because Primal Elements doesn't contain cinnamon oil; it contains ethylhexyl methoxycinnamate, which is a sunscreen. While the name sounds like cinnamon, it's not. Some people are sensitive to sunscreens, however, so you could look at the ingredients on other products you buy and see if you've used this one before.

## ICKY IRRITANTS?

What else? Well, menthol and camphor are mild irritants that could be causing the problem. And benzyl nicotinate is added to give your lips the tingling feeling that lip plumpers are supposed to provide. You might be reacting to that.

## SMELLS LIKE FRAGRANCE

Finally, fragrance is one of the usual suspects when it comes to skin reactions. The good news is that any lip plumper you try will probably have a different fragrance than Primal Elements. The rest of the formula seems unlikely to cause a problem.

## THE BOTTOM LINE

To be safe, look for a lip plumper that doesn't have ethyl methoxycinnamate, menthol, camphor or benzyl nicotinate, and that has a different fragrance.

# HOW MASCARA MAKES LASHES LOOK LOVELY

What's in mascara and how does it work? Here's the science-y scoop:

## HISTORY OF MASCARA

First, a quick bit of background: We know that mascaras have been around since at least 4000 BC because historical records show that Egyptians used charcoal and other minerals to darken their lashes and eyelids. In modern times, mascara first appeared in the form of a pressed cake that was applied by wetting a brush, rubbing it on the cake and then applying it to eyelashes. The cake consisted of a mixture of black pigments and soap chips. The next innovation in mascara involved a lotionlike version of the soap cake that was packaged in a tube and squeezed onto a small brush to apply. Mascara as we know it today was created in the 1960s with the invention of a grooved brush that could apply a consistent amount of the pigment. This is the basic form that's still used today.

## COMMON INGREDIENTS

The primary ingredients in mascara are pigments—the chemicals that provide color. Because U.S. federal regulations only allow certain colorants to be used in the area of the eye, only natural colors and inorganic pigments are used. Carbon black and iron oxides provide black, brown and red colors; ultramarine blue provides blue and green shades. These pigments are mixed together in a cosmetic base that is an emulsion of oils, waxes and water. For examples of these waxy ingredients, let's look at the ingredients list from Maybelline Great Lash:

> water, beeswax, ozokerite, shellac, glyceryl stearate, triethanolamine, propylene glycol, stearic acid, sorbitan sesquioleate, methylparaben, quaternium-15, quaternium-22, simethicone, butylparaben, iron oxides (may contain), titanium dioxide (may contain), ultramarine blue.

The beeswax, ozokerite, stearic acid and shellac provide the main body of the mascara and give it its waterproof and smudgeproof properties. Glyceryl stearate and triethanolamine are added to make sure the mascara can be washed off. The propylene glycol, sorbitan sesquioleate and simethicone, added as processing agents, help control the consistency of the product while methylparaben, quaternium-15, quaternium-22 and butylparaben are preservatives that keep the mascara free of "bugs." Finally, the iron oxides, titanium dioxide and ultramarine blue are the pigments.

## HOW MASCARA WORKS

This is really the simple part—when you stick the brush into the mascara tube and pull it out, a metering ring built into the orifice scrapes off the excess mascara so the brush has a controlled amount on it. When you brush your eyelashes, just the right amount gets delivered to each tiny hair fiber. The waxy nature of the mascara helps form a relatively thick coating that, due to the high wax concentration, is essentially waterproof. That's how a good mascara can resist smudging and bleeding. The result—your eyelashes get a nice splash of color and they look much plumper.

# SKEPTICAL ABOUT SMASHBOX'S O-GLOW

*Tamara's intrigued:* *Smashbox's O-Glow gel claims to generate a natural blushing effect by stimulating skin circulation. I'm intrigued, but the thought of intentionally inflaming my cheeks with a foreign substance strikes me as a bit weird. Does this really work?*

Let's take a look, shall we? According to Smashbox: "This revolutionary silicone-based clear gel works on every skin tone and is microcirculating and skin energizing to keep cheeks naturally flushed for hours." O-Glow does change to a pink color, but not for the reasons Smashbox gives us.

## EVERY PICTURE TELLS A STORY

O-Glow is a clear, colorless gel when it comes out of the tube. When rubbed on your cheek, it does turn from colorless to a lovely shade of pink. But is a "microcirculatory effect" really causing the color? The product changes color even when it's applied to a piece of white paper. Since paper doesn't have blood vessels, it's obvious that the effect has nothing to do with the circulatory system.

## HOW DOES IT REALLY WORK?

So how does it change color? Could it be the red dye #27 that's listed as one of the ingredients? Yep. We'll spare you the gory chemical details, but essentially the red dye is colorless when dissolved in a waterless base. When it comes in contact with moisture, the change in solubility and pH causes the dye to turn bright pink. That moisture can come from your skin, or even just the humidity in the air. So this product uses a dye to stain your cheeks, just like any other blush.

## THE BOTTOM LINE

While we appreciate the clever formulation work required to make a color-changing product, we say shame on Smashbox for presenting it in such a misleading way. It's a cool gimmick, but this product does *not* do what the company says it does. Considering how Smashbox marketers are blatantly misleading about this blush, we think they should be the ones with the red face!

# HOW DOES TUBING MASCARA WORK?

*Amanda asks:* I have recently purchased Blinc's Kiss Me Mascara. According to the company's product description, it works by "tubing" your lashes instead of "painting" them. It's beyond cool to take off my mascara at night and physically see it coming off in tubes from just "water and pressure," as the directions advise. Can you explain how it works?

## HAIRSPRAY IN A MASCARA

Unlike most mascaras, which are made with waxes, Blinc's Kiss Me is formulated with acrylate polymers. These polymers are similar to the ones used in hairsprays and they're what give Kiss Me its ability to form tiny tubes.

## TWO KINDS OF STRENGTH

When you apply any mascara to your lashes, you're coating the tiny hairs with a layer of product. When you try to remove the mascara, two factors come into play—cohesive strength (how well the mascara sticks to itself) and adhesive strength (how well it sticks to the eyelash).

## THE COOLNESS OF BLINC

Regular mascaras have a low cohesive strength and a relatively high adhesive strength. That means that when you try to remove regular mascaras they come off in little bits and pieces. Kiss Me mascara, on the other hand, has a high cohesive strength and a lower adhesive strength. Therefore, the mascara tends to stay in one piece as it slides off your lashes. That's why it looks like tiny tubes. That is cool!

## THE BOTTOM LINE

It's not your imagination and not a trick. Blinc's mascara is different from traditional mascaras because it uses a polymer instead of a wax.

# DOES FACIAL CLEANSER REALLY NEED TO BE APPLIED WITH AN "UPWARD MOTION"?

*Sherry says: On the back of my daily cleanser it instructs consumers to apply with an "upward motion." Is there any actual reason for this, or was it just thrown in to make the product seem more "special"? Should I be applying other products in a certain direction/motion?*

We aren't aware of any scientific need to apply facial cleansers with an upward motion. Our guess is that it's marketing-speak to make the cleanser sound more special. Maybe they think that since gravity drags your skin down (making it saggy and wrinkled) you can push your skin up to get rid of wrinkles. Who knows what they really mean.

## HOW YOU APPLY COSMETICS CAN MAKE A DIFFERENCE

Does your application technique ever make a difference? Yes, in some cases it does. Sunscreens, for example, need to be applied with very even, smooth strokes because they won't work very well if they don't evenly coat the skin. Same thing is true for sunless tanners—if you don't apply them evenly, you'll end up with streaks. Some types of makeup have similar application issues. For example, you need to be careful when applying wrinkle-concealing foundations to make sure they fill in those fine lines evenly.

## THE BOTTOM LINE

For some products, application technique does make a difference. That's not the case for facial cleansers. There's no technical reason that applying the product this way should help your skin. On the other hand, it won't hurt it, either.

# THE COLOR OF LOVE

The color red has long been associated with St. Valentine's Day. It's the color of the blood that runs through our hearts, so it's not surprising that it's always been linked to love and passion.

We see the color of passion reflected all over fashion and cosmetics. Everyone has (or should have!) a sexy red lipstick or nail polish for special romantic occasions. These products and many others exist thanks to the miracle of modern chemistry which has given us colorants such as FD&C red #40 and D&C red #33.

Of course, we weren't always lucky enough to have such a rainbow of reds to choose from. Originally, red dye came from a more natural, yet more disgusting, source: crushed insect bodies—the cochineal insect to be precise.

These bugs grow in certain varieties of cacti. They're hand-picked and immersed in hot water to kill them and to dissolve the waxy coating of their shells. The dead bugs are dried in the sun and then ground into a fine powder that can be used as dye for fabrics, foods and cosmetics.

Today, modern chemistry can synthetically create a wide variety of red dyes, so we don't have to rely on picking bugs off cacti to make our pucker look pretty. And that's just one more reason to be thankful to cosmetics chemists!

# HOW DOES EYELINER WORK?

Eyeliners are formulated into two basic types: pencils and liquids. While the details vary, both types use the same basic ingredients.

## BASE INGREDIENTS

The base is the backbone of the formula. In the case of pencils, it's the waxy/greasy matrix that forms the core of the pencil; in the liquids it's the water/oil emulsion in which the rest of the ingredients are suspended.

Typical base ingredients include waxes and oils, emollients (spreading agents) and, in the case of the liquid type, water and emulsifiers.

## COLORS

Colorants in eyeliners (and other cosmetics used around the eye) must be approved by the FDA (in the United States). Colorants that can be incorporated in products for other parts of the body aren't necessarily safe enough to be used around your eyes.

Typical colorants include iron oxides and ultramarine pigments. As discussed, carmine is another colorant you see from time to time. It's a red color made from crushed insect bodies. Mmmmm!

## CONTROL AGENTS

These are added to eyeliner formulations to make sure the product meets specifications when it's manufactured and that it maintains high quality. These include chemicals that control the pH, or acid/base balance of the product, and that keep the product free of bacteria and mold. In some oil-based formulas, an antioxidant may be added to keep the waxes and oils from going rancid.

Typical control agents include tocopherol (also known as vitamin E), used for its antioxidant properties, as well as citric acid, methylparaben, and propylparaben.

## FEATURED INGREDIENTS

Several things can be added to eyeliners to make them more appealing to consumers. These ingredients don't change the way the product works or the way it looks, but marketers add them because women think they are helpful. For some reason, aloe vera is a popular featured ingredient.

There are two ways that understanding eyeliner ingredients could be helpful. Let's say your favorite eyeliner is being discontinued. If you know what kind of base ingredients to look for, you might be able to pick a replacement without having to try so many new products. On the flip side, if you're experiencing irritation or an allergic reaction to your eyeliner, you might be able to figure out what ingredients to stay away from when you shop for a new one.

# SCIENTIFIC PROOF THAT MAKEUP REALLY HELPS

Many women spend countless hours a year putting on cosmetics and making sure they look just right before going out. Did you ever wonder if it was all worth it? Is the makeup really making you look that much more attractive? According to a team of psychologists in the United Kingdom, it is.

In their study, they found that men are more attracted to women with more color on their face. And they suggest that there is a good biological basis for this fact. They theorize that women with higher levels of estrogen naturally have more color than those with lower levels. And a higher level of estrogen is indicative of a more fertile woman. According to evolutionary theory, men should be inclined to find more fertile women more attractive.

The experiment involved measuring hormone levels of a group of volunteer women and then having those women rated for attractiveness by another group of both men and women. It turns out that the ones who were rated highest in attractiveness were also the ones who had the highest level of estrogen.

Of course, you probably didn't need a scientific study to validate the use of makeup. People discovered the benefits centuries ago. But we here at the Beauty Brains are happy to know that it isn't all just a waste of time. And it's also nice to know that the chosen career of the Brains is playing a crucial role in the noble quest of successfully propagating a diverse population.

# WHY IS THERE BORAX IN LUSH LIP BALMS?

**Debby wants to know:** *I read a discussion on the internet about the use of sodium borate in some of the lip balms from Lush. Could you tell me something more about this ingredient?*

A lot of people ask us if Lush formulas are really different than mass market products. In this case, they are.

## WHAT IS BORAX?

Sodium borate, also called borax, is used in products that contain high levels of beeswax. The borax reacts with the beeswax to form an emulsion, a stable mixture of oil and water.

## HOW IS LUSH DIFFERENT THAN OTHER PRODUCTS?

Most emulsions, like your typical skin lotion, are "oil in water" emulsions, which means that the oil drops are dispersed in the water. Borax-beeswax emulsions are unusual—they're "water in oil" emulsions, so the water drops are dispersed in the oil. That type of emulsion tends to be more waterproof, which is good for a lip balm. Also, because the borax-beeswax combination forms a stable emulsion without the help of additional emulsifiers, this type of formula supports Lush's position of not using excessive chemicals.

## IS BORAX SAFE?

And a final note: If you do any kind of web search on borax, you'll find that it can also be used as an insecticide, but don't worry about that. It's only toxic to humans at very high levels—in fact, it has the same toxicity profile as common table salt. So a little bit in your lip balm is perfectly fine.

## THE BOTTOM LINE

Sodium borate is a naturally derived useful cosmetic ingredient that helps make beeswax lipbalm work better.

# CAN LIP GLOSS HELP YOU LOSE WEIGHT?

*Alicia asks:* I've heard about a lip gloss called Promise from Omega Tech Labs that is supposed to have weight-loss benefits. Can this really be true?

## APPETITE SUPPRESSANT IN LIP GLOSS

According to the company, the lip gloss contains a blend of botanical oils (castor oil, coconut oil and evening primrose oil) that works as an appetite suppressant. Experts say that these ingredients can work, but they don't believe you will get enough exposure from the lip gloss to make much difference.

## SMELLS CAN HELP YOU SLIM DOWN

While we are highly skeptical, there is some science backing up the concept behind this product. Researchers at the Smell & Taste Treatment and Research Foundation have done studies showing that odors can actually help people lose weight. If Promise lip gloss contains appetite suppressant oils and odors that help curb your appetite, it might have such an effect.

## COULD BE TOO TASTY

On the other hand, the flavor could actually stimulate your appetite and have the opposite effect! Since the company offers no clinical study to support its claims, we can't know for sure whether it works. But, hey, it's worth a try. It's probably a good lip gloss and if it has the added benefit of helping you lose weight without taking another spinning class, how cool is that?

## THE BOTTOM LINE

We doubt that a lip gloss will have any significant impact on your weight. Feel free to try it, but if you want weight loss be sure to eat fewer calories and exercise.

# WHY WOMEN USE MAKEUP

Most women will say that they use makeup to look and feel prettier. But an interesting study from the *Journal of Cosmetic Science* digs a little deeper. According to researchers in France, makeup stimulates three of our senses. First, it stimulates the sense of sight because of the visual impact of the pretty colors we smear all over our eyes, lips and cheeks. Second, depending on the kind of makeup we use, it can also stimulate our sense of smell. Third, makeup also stimulates our sense of touch. That happens during the application process or long after the product has been applied. The study also raised the intriguing notion that makeup can stimulate not only our hands and fingers, but also all our body surfaces.

But the most interesting aspect of this study was the way it tried to understand why we like makeup so much. The researchers say that makeup's effect on our senses results in two different psychological effects—camouflage and seduction.

Camouflage is all about reducing anxiety, supporting our internal defense mechanisms and promoting emotional stability. Seduction is about being more socially assertive and extroverted. The way you use makeup depends on your individual psychological profile.

# CAN SMASHBOX HALO POWDER HYDRATE YOUR SKIN?

*Tonya says:* I've heard about Smashbox Halo, a new powder that claims to hydrate your skin with encapsulated water and also prevent aging by using gogi berries as an antioxidant. Can your skin actually absorb anything from your foundation? If you use a primer as a "barrier," doesn't that defeat the purpose of this product? How can you encapsulate water in a pressed powder that is then shaved to produce a loose powder? Reviewers say that their skin feels hydrated, but the product description only says that the water gives a hydrated appearance. Is this all marketing hype?

While Smashbox makes good products, it's our opinion that they, like many other cosmetic companies, tend to exaggerate the benefits of their technology (see page 112 for our discussion of O-Glow cheek color). Smashbox Halo seems no different.

## POWDERED WATER
The idea of "encapsulated water" is cool, but it's not a new concept and it wasn't invented by Smashbox. It's a simple matter of mixing water with fumed silica under high shear conditions. The tiny silica particles coat the water droplets, creating tiny water capsules. When you rub the powder, the capsules break and water is released. The cooling effect you feel as the water is released could provide the hydrated feeling that you asked about, but it's not enough to provide a true moisturizing effect. To really hydrate skin, you need to add not only water but also an occlusive film that will prevent moisture from evaporating. The discrete particles in a powder can't be as effective as a uniform film.

## THE BOTTOM LINE
This product may be a perfectly fine powder but the hydration claim is just a cool gimmick that doesn't add much benefit.

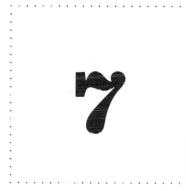

# 7 NAIL KNOWLEDGE

From putting polish on to taking it off, this chapter is chock-full of nail knowledge you need. We'll give you scientific tips to follow for longer, stronger nails and we'll tell you five ways to avoid ruining your nails. (We'll even explain how *not* to get ripped off by your nail salon.) If you've ever worried about breathing nail polish fumes or wondered why your polish can turn your nails yellow, this is info you'll need to read!

# CAN UV NAIL POLISH DRYERS DAMAGE SKIN?

*Jeanne is jittery:* My nail salon uses a UV nail polish dryer. Should I be worried about getting age spots on the top of my hands and feet from the UV light?

We looked into UV dryers and found that the wavelength of the light they produce *is* the same type that causes photoaging and skin cancer. (That's the UVA range from about 320 nm to 400 nm for those of you keeping score at home.)

## NAIL DRYERS WON'T CAUSE SUNBURN

Fortunately, the danger seems pretty slight because drying lamps have a very low power output—only around 10 watts. Compare that to the power of a full-sized tanning bed that can put out up to 2,400 watts! So your fingers probably aren't in much danger. Still, if you're concerned, you could apply some sunblock before using the lamp.

## BUT THEY CAN STILL BE DANGEROUS

So is there *any* danger associated with using UV drying lamps? Yes, in fact, you might be in danger of getting ripped off!

That's because UV light only works on special, more expensive, topcoats that contain a certain type of acrylic polymer that is cross-linked by the light. Some salons try to save money by using a regular topcoat before using the drying lamp. The UV light won't do anything to make that kind of polish dry faster. So whether you use OPI, Sally Hansen or any other brand, it makes sense to ask what topcoat the nail technician is using so you can make sure you're getting what you pay for!

## THE BOTTOM LINE

There is no evidence that the light from UV dryers will damage your skin, but you might want to apply sunscreen just in case.

# FIVE WAYS TO RUIN YOUR FINGERNAILS

*Diane's in digit danger:* My fingernails go through seasonal cycles. Sometimes they are long, strong and healthy. At other times they split and bend and look ragged. I've used Sally Hansen's Maximum Growth, but it doesn't seem to do much. Got any ideas? Also, why does Sally Hansen have so many products that all seem to do the same thing (i.e., Hard As Nails, Maximum Growth, etc.)?

It's hard to say for sure what the seasonal changes are that you're experiencing, but many things can affect the condition of your nails.

Here are our top five finger factors that can make your nails look hammered.

**1 Excessive environmental dryness**
Are your nails worse in the winter? If your nail condition is literally changing with the seasons, it may be due to humidity. Nails, like skin, are subject to the drying effects of the environment. *Solution:* If your nails are dry and raggedy in the winter, use more lotion.

**2 Hyper hand washing**
Does your job (or hobby or home life) cause you to wash your hands on some occasions more than others? Washing your hands with soap and water can dry out nails. That could be causing an apparent seasonal change. *Solution:* Use a mild hand wash instead of bar soap and don't skimp on the lotion.

**3 Damage from drying solvents**
Are you engaged in any activities that would expose your nails to solvents? For example, home repair projects (like painting a room or varnishing wood trim) could be seasonal activities that negatively impact the condition of your nails. *Solution:* Hire someone else to handle these projects or wear protective gloves.

**4 Negative nail product usage**
Do you occasionally use nail-hardening products? Since you asked about several Sally Hansen products, I'm guessing you do. Those products do make nails harder but they can also make them brittle and more prone to breaking. That's because they use a chemical called formaldehyde to cross-link the keratin protein in nails. *Solution:* Skip the hardeners and see if it helps. (And to answer your question about why they have so many products that seem to do the same thing, we have one word: capitalism.)

# 5 The horrible heartbreak of psoriasis

Psoriasis is a disease that causes your skin to become red and scaly. About half the people who suffer from this condition also have nail problems, particularly pitting, rippling and/or splitting of the nail. *Solution:* If you think psoriasis might be responsible for your nail problems, check with a dermatologist for treatment options.

## THE BOTTOM LINE

No cosmetic will make your nails grow longer and stronger, but you can do things to improve their condition, like applying moisturizing lotion, using mild detergents, using rubber gloves when doing dishes, skipping the top coat and treating your psoriasis.

# ARE NAIL POLISH FUMES DANGEROUS?

*Loretta breathes this question:* Is inhaling nail polish fumes harmful if you're exposed to them for about thirty minutes or so per week?

Nearly all the popular brands of nail polish contain organic solvents and methacrylates. The March 2002 issue of *Neuropsychiatry, Neuropsychology, and Behavioral Neurology* summarizes a study by Gina LaSasso, PhD, et al, that shows that prolonged exposure to nail polish fumes can affect the way your brain works.

The researchers tested thirty-three nail-salon technicians, and compared them to the same number of demographically similar control subjects (in other words, women from the same socioeconomic group who had no exposure to nail polish or other toxic chemicals). Both groups were given a series of psychological, neuropsychological and neurosensory tests.

## NAIL POLISH FUMES AFFECT BRAIN FUNCTIONS

Their study showed three main results:

1. The nail technicians performed statistically worse than the control group on tests that measured attention and brain processing speed.
2. The nail technicians and the control group showed no statistical differences in learning and memory, fine motor coordination or on measures of depression and anxiety.
3. The nail technicians' sense of smell was statistically worse than the control group's.

## FRESH AIR, NOT FUMES

What does all this mean? Apparently, exposure to enough nail polish fumes can make your brain a little slow and fuzzy. Kinda scary, huh? Unfortunately, the study didn't provide details on how long this effect lasts, so we don't know if your brain returns to normal once you've gotten away from the nail fumes.

And while the study did measure the size of the salon, the amount of ventilation and the number of hours that the technicians worked, the data can't be used to predict what would happen at a lower exposure. In other words, if you're in a nail salon long enough, you may experience these problems. But is thirty minutes a week enough to cause an effect? It doesn't look like it, but clearly more studies are needed.

## THE BOTTOM LINE

It's not very likely that you will die from inhaling nail polish fumes thirty minutes a week, but make sure you get plenty of fresh air when you're getting your nails done.

# WHY DOES NAIL POLISH REMOVER STOP WORKING?

*Izzy wants to know:* What happened to my polish remover? I use Cutex and now it takes forever to get the polish off.

Our guess is that you might have accidentally bought the wrong Cutex! Basically, there are two different kinds of nail polish removers: acetone and non-acetone. They work by dissolving the hard film that's left on your nails by the ingredients in the polish.

## ACETONE

Acetone is a very powerful solvent and it's hands down the best at removing polish. But it's also very harsh because it removes a lot of natural oils from your skin. In fact, sometimes your skin will look really white if you've used too much acetone on it. That means you've dried it out.

## NON-ACETONE

Non-acetone removers use less aggressive solvents, like ethyl acetate and isopropyl alcohol. They also add moisturizing agents to overcome the drying effect. However, these formulations don't dissolve the polish coating as efficiently, so you'll have to work harder to take off all the old color.

## THE BOTTOM LINE

To please all consumers, many nail polish remover brands, like Cutex, make both acetone and non-acetone products. Just be careful to read the label so you know which one you're getting! If you prefer a powerful polish remover, look for acetone on the ingredients list and stay away from products that are non-acetone or acetone-free.

# WHY DOES WEARING POLISH TURN YOUR NAILS YELLOW?

*Sue wonders: Why does wearing nail polish turn my nails yellow? Also, is there anything I can do to prevent it?*

Nail polish can turn your nails yellow. There are a few reasons for this.

## COLOR REACTION

Some of the darker-colored polishes can stain nails due to a chemical reaction between the colorant and the nail plate. This reaction is hard to predict because it doesn't happen for everybody or for every dark color. It can also take a few days to a few weeks to occur.

## FORMALDEHYDE

It's also possible that formaldehyde (one of the ingredients in many nail polishes) is causing the problem. This chemical can react with the keratin protein in your nails and make them brittle and yellow.

## MEDICAL ISSUES

Finally, if your nails are really yellowed and disfigured, you may have a nail infection or a more serious medical condition known as Yellow Nail Syndrome. So what can you do to keep polish from turning your nails yellow? Read on!

## TIPS FOR AVOIDING YELLOW NAILS

1. Don't try to scrape off the stained area because it will damage and weaken the nail.

2. Stay away from dark polish colors (which will greatly reduce your fashion options).

3. Wear a base coat to protect your nails from staining (this makes sense to us).

4. Look for nail polishes that don't have formaldehyde in the ingredients list. (There's no guarantee that this will work but, hey, it beats this next tip we found from one of the nail polish companies.)

5. Wear gloves (now there's a practical idea!).

6. Stop wearing polish and wait for your nails to grow out. (Also not too practical; this could take four to six months.)

7. Soak your nails in ½ cup of water and the juice of one lemon for up to 15 minutes, once a week, according to Sally Hansen. (We're skeptical about this one, but you can always add some sugar and just drink it as lemonade.)

8. Buy only yellow shades of polish so you can't tell if your nails are stained or not (just kidding).

## THE BOTTOM LINE

Nail polish can stain your nails yellow, but by choosing the right shades, using a protective base coat and wearing gloves, you should be able to control the problem.

# FOUR EASY TIPS FOR LONGER, STRONGER NAILS

*Willie wants to know:* I've stopped biting my nails and now I'm trying to grow them out. However, after they reach a certain length they start to break. I've been using a nail hardener to no avail! Are there any nail products that you could recommend that could promote stronger nails?

The idea that nail hardeners can help your nails grow longer is a myth, but here are four things you *can* do to help improve your nails:

**1** **Avoid nail polishes containing formaldehyde.**
This ingredient can chemically react with the keratin protein in your nails. While

it does make the nails harder, it also makes them so stiff that they become brittle so they actually break *more* easily.

## 2 Don't bother with gelatin.
Many products claim that gelatin strengthens nails because it is made from protein, but there is no scientific evidence that gelatin has any benefit to nails.

## 3 Limit your use of polish removers.
These products contain alcohol and other solvents that dry nails out, making them more prone to breakage.

## 4 Use a good hand cream or cuticle cream.
Daily exposure to detergents and harsh chemicals dries out your nails and makes them break more easily. By moisturizing them often, you can prevent loss of moisture and reduce the chance of breakage. Lotions with petrolatum or mineral oil are the best.

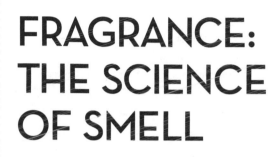

# 8 FRAGRANCE: THE SCIENCE OF SMELL

Have you ever wondered why perfumes smell so good? Then you'll love learning about "Living Flower Technology" and the basic chemistry of how fragrances work. We'll also explain why some scents seem to last and last while others disappear in no time. And along the way we'll bust a few myths about fragrances.

# WHAT MAKES SOME PERFUMES LAST SO LONG?

*Jansen needs justification:* I am currently using an eau de parfum called Allure Homme Sport by Chanel, and it is the most long-lasting fragrance ever. (And, yes, I am a bloke.) One of my chemist friends told me that this has to do with the exclusive alcohol that Chanel uses in its perfumes; it probably has a low boiling point, so the fragrances are more volatile. I wonder: How true is this statement?

While we chemists usually stick together, we have to disagree with your friend's assessment of why Allure lasts so long. To explain why, here's a quick lesson on fragrance chemistry.

Fragrances are complex mixtures of natural and synthetic chemicals designed to create a specific scent. The fragrance ingredients are mixed with alcohol (specifically ethanol) to dilute them to a usable level. Ethanol is used because it's safe, it's a good solvent and it evaporates quickly. In fact, the alcohol is the *first* thing that evaporates. That's why when you first spray on perfume you want to wait a few seconds before smelling it. Otherwise, you get a nose full of sharp alcohol odor. As the alcohol flashes off, the other ingredients in the fragrance are more noticeable; these ingredients are loosely grouped into three categories, depending on how fast they evaporate.

## THREE NOTES

**Top notes** evaporate quickly so you smell them first. These tend to be lighter in nature—think citrus-type scents. They are also the first notes to wear out over the course of the day.

**Middle notes** evaporate a bit more slowly and create the body of the fragrance; these are usually a combination of floral and/or fruity notes.

**Bottom notes** are the heavier, longer-lasting fragrance components. Perfumers describe these notes with terms like woody, balsamic, smoky or musky. These notes are the "anchors" that help the fragrance last longer. Bingo!

## THE BOTTOM LINE

Allure lasts longer because of the bottom notes in the fragrance not because of the alcohol. And speaking of alcohol, tell your chemist friend he or she should buy you a cocktail to make up for the bad advice!

# CAN THE FRAGRANCE ADDED TO LOTIONS DAMAGE SKIN?

**Mary asks:** *Are the flowery scents in body lotion or shampoos harmful in any way?*

With all the advice and advertising encouraging people to avoid fragrances, you might wonder why beauty product manufacturers keep making fragranced products and why people keep buying them. The simple answer is because that's what people want and, for the vast majority of consumers, fragrances in products are not harmful. Pleasant odors help improve the product experience and people often buy products just because they love the scent. It's clear that fragranced products are here to stay

## YES, FOR SOME PEOPLE

However, flowery scents aren't for everyone. In a recent study published in the *British Journal of Dermatology*, an average of 2.3 percent of adults had allergic reactions to fragrance chemicals when exposed to patch testing. Adverse fragrance reactions include skin problems like contact dermatitis and skin photosensitivity, and respiratory problems. Over 100 fragrance ingredients have been identified as allergens. The main sensitizers include cinnamic aldehyde, oak moss and isoeugenol. It's interesting to us that all three of these compounds are "natural"

## FRAGRANCE-FREE IS A GOOD OPTION IF YOU NEED IT

If you are allergic to certain fragrance compounds, then your best bet is to use fragrance-free products. In the United States, companies are now required to list fragrance allergens on their labels. If you know you are allergic to a specific compound, then look for it on labels and avoid those products.

## UNSCENTED IS NOT THE SAME AS FRAGRANCE-FREE

One word of caution is that *unscented* products are not the same as *fragrance-free*. Often an unscented product will contain a fragrance that is designed to offset the base odor of the formula. Your nose may not realize the product contains a fragrance, but if you are allergic to any of the compounds in the fragrance, your body won't be fooled. Fragrance-free products contain no fragrance and are the safest if you are trying to avoid fragrance chemicals.

## THE BOTTOM LINE

Fragrances in cosmetics and personal care products can be harmful to some people but are not harmful for the majority of the population. If you suspect that you are allergic or are concerned about fragrances, you should avoid them. Most people prefer products that smell nice, but a good odor is not needed for them to work.

# ARE PERFUMES MADE FROM NATURAL INGREDIENTS?

*Deborah asks:* Are perfumes made from real flowers or fake chemicals?

Perfumes are made with a mixture of natural and synthetic ingredients, and one of the most interesting approaches to creating synthetic ingredients involves capturing the scent that a living flower exudes.

### POWERFUL PERFUME

Perfume is wonderful, but nothing smells quite as nice as a fresh-cut flower. Or does it? Is it possible that modern science can make a perfume that smells just like a real flower? The answer is yes! Scientists at International Flavors and Fragrance (IFF), one of the world's largest fragrance companies, have developed a new technology that allows them to reproduce the *exact* scent of a living flower—without even having to pick it.

Floral fragrance ingredients were originally created by picking a flower and processing it to extract the chemical components responsible for its aroma. While this process did isolate some of the chemicals responsible for the flower's smell, it did not capture the *exact* same scent molecules that were released by the flower and picked up by your nose. That's because a living flower releases different chemicals than a dead, cut flower. Therefore, it was really impossible to replicate the exact scent of fresh flowers.

### LIVING FLOWER TECHNOLOGY

But IFF's new Living Flower head-space analysis technology changes all that. No, head-space analysis does not refer to some kind of psychoanalytical technique. It's a way of collecting the scent of a living, growing flower, instead of just extracting chemicals from a dead flower.

It works like this: A large glass globe is placed around the living flower to capture the scent it releases. This globe is connected to a sophisticated gas chromatograph that analyzes the exact composition of the scent. Chemists then use this analysis as a road map to create a synthetic chemical that smells exactly like the original. (This same technique can be applied to fruits as well as flowers.) So instead of chopping up dead flowers, scientists can now create more natural-smelling perfumes from living plants. It's another great example of better living through chemistry.

## THE BOTTOM LINE

In our opinion, the best products take something from nature and improve on it. And that's how Living Flower technology works.

# IS IT SAFE TO SPRAY PERFUME ON YOUR HAIR?

*Jo just wants to know:* My girlfriends and I were having a discussion about hair, and I mentioned that I like to spray some perfume on my hair, as I prefer my locks to be scented. My friends tell me this is terrible thing to do, as the alcohol in perfume will dry out my hair. Is there any truth to that, or can I keep on spritzing?

You're lucky to have friends who are so concerned about the health of your hair. But in this particular case we'd have to say their concerns are largely unfounded.

## ALCOHOL ANXIETY

- Yes it's true that alcohol can be drying to the hair and skin. That's because alcohol can dissolve, and therefore rearrange the natural oils in your hair and skin that provide a moisture barrier. If you remove the oils, the water can evaporate more quickly. But for this to happen you almost need to submerge hair in alcohol; a small amount of alcohol that evaporates quickly will not have a significant effect.

- Perfume does contain alcohol, but not enough to "submerge," or totally saturate, hair fibers. By way of comparison, consider hairspray. Aerosol hairsprays contain up to 50% alcohol and are sprayed for four or five seconds. Given that most hairsprays deliver a few tenths of a gram of product for every second they are sprayed, this means that hairsprays deliver several grams of alcohol to your hair each time you style your hair. Perfumes, on the other hand, have a higher concentration of alcohol (about 90%), but a spritz or two only delivers a fraction of a gram to your hair. So you're probably putting about two to three times more alcohol on your hair from hairspray than from perfume.

- Whatever alcohol that is deposited on your hair evaporates very quickly so small amounts (less than a gram, as we just discussed) spread over a large surface area (your hairstyle) means that there's not a lot of alcohol sitting on your hair for a long period. Therefore, there's very little chance that it will dry out your hair.

## THE BOTTOM LINE

Your friends are right that *lots* of alcohol is bad for your hair (and for your liver as well). But small amounts spritzed on occasionally will have little effect on the overall condition of your hair.

# CAN PHEROMONE FRAGRANCES GET YOU A DATE?

**Ann asks:** *Do pheromone fragrances really attract the opposite sex?*

Could a chemical actually improve your sex life? Yes, if the results of a study by San Francisco State University researchers are accurate. According to their work, men are more attracted to women wearing pheromones, resulting in more dates, kisses, cuddles and even sex.

## WHAT ARE PHEROMONES?

Pheromones are a type of compound that allow animals to chemically communicate with each other. They are versatile chemicals that help ants figure out how to get home, that let dogs mark their territory and that let other mammals know when to mate. The word *pheromone* comes from the Greek words *pherin*, meaning to transfer, and *hormon*, meaning to excite. These chemicals are similar to hormones but instead of working within the body, they work between bodies. The chemical communication of pheromones is simple. One animal (or human) releases the pheromone and another senses it. In essence, the behavior of the sensing animal is controlled by the pheromone releaser. In mammals, pheromones are detected by an organ called the vomeronasal organ (VMO), which is located somewhere in the head between the nose and mouth. Pheromones are a bit like odor molecules, but they have a much different effect.

## DO PHEROMONES REALLY WORK?

Well, if pheromones really worked it would mean that controlling the behavior of people would be simple. If you wanted someone to fall in love with you, you could simply spray some pheromones whenever that person is around. Fortunately, human behavior is a bit more complicated than that.

It is still debated among scientists whether pheromones have an effect or not. These researchers demonstrated that women actually saw an increase in sociosexual activity when wearing perfume that contained pheromones. The impressive part of this research was that it was compared to a placebo control. But one study (of thirty-six women) isn't enough to substantiate these incredible claims.

Other researchers have looked at all the human pheromone data and the results are inconclusive. Yes, pheromones are real. Yes, they have some physiological effect (such as synchronizing women's menstrual cycles). But how much pheromones change behavior is still unclear.

## THE BOTTOM LINE

We're not saying these products will definitely work. But they might just be the thing that helps make your next date more memorable!

# CAN PERFUME MAKE YOU THINNER?

**Erica asks:** *I know this is a crazy question, but are there any cosmetics that help with dieting?*

By legal definition, cosmetics can only "beautify" your body. If they have a physiological effect, then they are classified as a drug. But we did find an interesting fragrance study by Dr. Allen Hirsch and his team at the Smell & Taste Treatment and Research Foundation which shows that the *perception* of body weight could be affected by the fragrance you wear.

## LOSE POUNDS WITH PERFUME

In the study, four groups of about fifty men each looked at a woman (actual stats: 5'9"; 245 pounds) and estimated how much she weighed. For three of the groups, the woman was wearing one of three different fragrances (citrus floral, sweet pea/lily of the valley or floral/spicy). For the fourth group, the woman wore no fragrance.

The researchers then compared the weight estimates of each group for differences. Surprisingly, when the woman wore the floral/spicy fragrance, the men estimated her weight to be four pounds less than her actual weight. And if the guys liked the fragrance, they said she looked a full twelve pounds less! Without a single sit-up being done.

## THE BOTTOM LINE

Now, this research seems a little weak for us science-minded Beauty Brains, but it is certainly provocative. And even if the results can't be duplicated, it couldn't hurt to start wearing a floral and spice fragrance. I mean, wouldn't you want to spray on a fragrance and look like you'd lost some weight?

# WHAT'S THE RELATIONSHIP BETWEEN QUALITY AND PRICE WHEN IT COMES TO FRAGRANCE?

*Carla's quandary: Does the quality or amount of perfume/fragrance in a personal care product affect its price? I've noticed that some of the more expensive ones are more pleasantly fragrant than those that are cheaper, even though they are somewhat similar in ingredients.*

Carla's got a nose for the truth, as fragrance can be the single most costly ingredient in some formulas.

This is not true for makeup products like lipstick, blush and eye shadow, which typically contain only small amounts of masking fragrance. It's also not typically true for high-end skin treatments that contain expensive active ingredients like hyaluronic acid or retinoid derivatives. But for shampoos, body washes and other products that deliver a "fragrance experience," the scent can add a pretty penny to the final product cost.

### THE FRAGRANCE EQUATION

Formulators look at two variables when factoring in the fragrance cost—the cost of the fragrance itself and how much of the fragrance is used in the finished product. Let's look at cost first. A cheap fragrance can cost as little as $4 or $5 per pound, while an expensive one can cost $20 per pound or more. Spending more on a fragrance gives the perfumers more latitude in which ingredients they can use.

Perfumers can make a very cheap-smelling lemon fragrance (think furniture polish) for a couple of bucks per pound. For more money, they can make it smell as sweet as summertime lemonade.

Next, consider the concentration, which is how much fragrance is used in the finished product. We'll use body wash as example. In a "regular" (i.e., "cheap") body wash, the fragrance concentration can be as low as half a percent (0.5%). But for a luscious, fill-up-your-bath-stay-on-your-skin-all-day kind of fragrance, the formula may need to contain as much as 2–5% fragrance.

## DOLLARS AND SCENTS

Now let's do the math on the cost. The cheap body wash (using a cheap $4 per pound fragrance at 0.5%) only contains $.02 worth of fragrance per pound of body wash. (A fifteen-ounce bottle is slightly less than one pound.) On the other hand, the luscious body wash (using a $15 per pound fragrance at 5.0%) contains $.75 of fragrance! Considering that all the other ingredients in the body wash could cost somewhere between $.25 and $.50, that's a lot!

## THE BOTTOM LINE

In general, manufacturers of more expensive products spend more on fragrance. For an indulgent product like a yummy bubble bath, that could be money well spent. But if the product is purely functional (like a bar of soap) you might want to shop around for a less expensive alternative.

# CAN AROMATHERAPY HELP YOU SLEEP?

*Kay's question:* *In my Greek mythology class we just read about the myth of Psyche who traveled to Hell to bring back Persephone's makeup box. When she opened the box, according to the story, the cosmetics inside made her fall asleep. That sounds like modern-day aromatherapy! Is it possible to formulate a product that can really do that?*

We love the myth of Psyche (who happened to be married to Cupid, by the way!). Fortunately for them, the story doesn't end there because Psyche eventually woke up and they lived happily ever after. While it's nice to see true love triumph, the myth does leave a nagging question for us science types: Can cosmetics really relax you enough to make you fall asleep? Believe it or not, modern science suggests that this may actually be possible.

## DOES AROMATHERAPY REALLY WORK?

According to an article in the April 2004 Issue of *Natural Health,* Namni Goel, PhD, an assistant professor of psychology and neuroscience at Wesleyan University conducted a study that indicates that smelling lavender oil can make you sleep more deeply.

This study involved fifteen women and ten men who were asked to intermittently sniff one of two vials for thirty minutes before sleep. One vial contained lavender oil, the other contained an odorless control (the panelists were told this might be a scent diluted so much that it was undetectable). Then, using electrodes, Goel measured the sleeping panelists' brain waves.

The results showed that the panelists who sniffed lavender oil had significantly increased slow-wave sleep brain patterns, which are indicative of a very deep stage of sleep. While this research doesn't mean that lavender can replace sleeping pills, it does indicate there may be a valid scientific basis for some aromatherapy claims.

## THE BOTTOM LINE

Our understanding of the effects of fragrance on the brain are far from complete, but it does appear that in some cases there is an interaction. Just beware of products that make bogus aromatherapy claims that aren't backed up by science.

# PART IV

# THE BEAUTY INDUSTRY

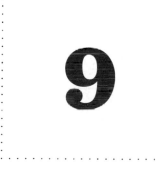

# SCANDALS AND SECRETS OF THE BEAUTY BIZ

Believe it or not, beauty companies stretch the truth once in a while to entice you to buy products. We'll tell you all about their "dirty secrets" so you can tell when they're promising more than their products can deliver and when you're paying more than you probably should. We'll even explain the true meaning of confusing buzzwords that you hear every day, like *natural* and *organic*.

# THE THREE BIGGEST FIBS THAT COSMETICS COMPANIES TELL

**Kris's question:** *My mother-in-law is a "beauty consultant" for a company called BeautiControl and they seem to have a pretty extensive line of skin care products. Do you know anything about the quality of this line and/or can you recommend any BeautiControl products?*

Based on what we've seen, BeautiControl products seem to be of reasonable quality. They're also very pricey, but if you can afford them, that's your decision.

What bugs us, and the reason that we would not recommend them, is the way the company hypes its products. We understand the need for creative marketing, but when a company makes statements that border on being false, that really disturbs us. We just hate being mislead and we *really* hate it under the guise of science. There are at least three tip-offs when a company is stretching the truth about its products. Here are some examples using BeautiControl.

## 1. CLAIMS OF EXCLUSIVITY
*What's misleading?*
BeautiControl says that "only" its products can give you a certain benefit.

*What's the truth?*
The truth is, unless the company has a patent or a documented trade secret, BeautiControl is using the same technology as everyone else in the industry.

*What's the example?*
BeautiControl says, "Only BeautiControl offers comprehensive, customized skin care that addresses what your skin needs when it needs it." Based on its product catalog, the company appears to have typical cleansers, toners, lotions and the like that are offered by many, many other companies. So why does the literature say that "only" BeautiControl offers this kind of treatment?

## 2. IMPLYING SUPERIOR PERFORMANCE WITHOUT SUBSTANTIATION
*What's misleading?*
BeautiControl marketers tell you their products work better than anyone else's.

*What's the truth?*
If they make claims like that, they'd better have some kind of proof.

*What's the example?*

BeautiControl says, "Far beyond traditional dry, combination and oily skin care, BeautiControl takes an innovative, personal approach to provide total skin wellness through…" Blah, blah, blah. Again, with conventional products there is no way they can convince us that their products are "far beyond traditional" ones. Yes, they may be applying a different marketing spin, but there is no technology muscle behind their mouth.

## 3. "MAGIC" INGREDIENT CLAIMS

*What's misleading?*

They say that some sexy-sounding ingredient makes the product work.

*What's the truth?*

In reality, most of the time it's the formula as a whole and not any single ingredient that makes the product work.

*What's the example?*

BeautiControl says one of its products is "formulated with the rejuvenating minerals of the Dead Sea." Minerals don't rejuvenate skin; moisturizing agents do.

OK, technically BeautiControl isn't "lying" to us, but their public relations department is certainly overstating the uniqueness of their line. And as scientists, that kind of hype turns us off.

## THE BOTTOM LINE

Most beauty companies in the United States produce high-quality products that will provide basic benefits like cleansing, moisturizing and otherwise beautifying. Unfortunately, the claims they make are often exaggerations of what you'll really experience.

# WHAT DOES *ORGANIC* REALLY MEAN?

*Stacey says:* I'm confused by all the companies that sell organic and natural products. What makes a product organic?

For chemists like the Beauty Brains, the meaning of *organic* is clear. It is any chemical compound that contains carbon. In fact, to get a college chemistry degree, you take a year of organic chemistry, in which you memorize endless chemical reactions between hydrocarbons, oxygen, nitrogen and more. Many a chemist wannabe switched to a marketing major after flunking organic chemistry.

## WHAT DOES *ORGANIC* MEAN IN TERMS OF COSMETICS?

*Organic* doesn't mean quite the same thing in the cosmetics industry as it does in the food industry. To consumers it can mean "natural," "green," "chemical-free" or "found at Whole Foods." But there is no cosmetics industry-standard meaning for terms like *organic* or *natural*. Unlike the farming industry, these terms are not regulated for cosmetics. Companies can pretty much claim that anything is natural or organic.

For example, imagine a body wash formula. It contains all kinds of synthetic surfactants, fragrances, preservatives and colors. But it also contains 85–90 percent water. A company might simply claim "90 percent organic" or "90 percent natural" and be telling the truth. Certainly, this isn't in the spirit of what people believe *organic* to mean, but it is within the law.

The people at Burt's Bees are outraged by the tricks some companies are playing on the public. They are campaigning to get tighter regulations on cosmetics that use terms such as *natural* or *organic*. Stay tuned to see if they will make a difference.

## ARE ORGANIC PRODUCTS BETTER?

Incidentally, natural or organic cosmetic products don't provide any added benefit for consumers. In fact companies that strive to make *organic* or *natural* products often end up with finished products that are functionally inferior to more mainstream products. This is the real trade-off when it comes to natural or organic products. That and a hugely higher cost for an inferior product.

Remember, cosmetics are not food. No one has ever proven there is a benefit to "organically" derived cosmetics.

## THE BOTTOM LINE

Organic is a term used by chemists to describe carbon-containing molecules. And it's used by cosmetic marketers to trick you into buying cosmetics that are often functionally inferior.

# 5 HOME BEAUTY GADGETS THAT REALLY WORK

While there are a lot of products out there making false claims about what they can do, there are several new beauty gadgets on the market that do work. According to Dr. Thomas Rohrer, MD, clinical associate professor of dermatology at Boston University Medical Center, "We are getting to the point where, for certain things, patients may be able to treat themselves safely and fairly effectively at home."

However, Dr. Rohrer also points out that these treatments are still less effective than the devices used by physicians: "They're not going to be nearly as powerful" but "they may be effective enough…to improve some conditions." Here are five beauty gadgets that Dr. Rohrer says really work:

**1. Hair removal:** *The Epila SI-808 laser and the Spa Touch from Radiancy*
According to Dr. Rohrer, Spa Touch showed moderate efficacy with patients reporting an average 66% reduction in unwanted hair counts. At nine months' follow-up, patients noted about a one-third reduction. Furthermore, there were minimal side effects.

**2. Hair growth:** *HairMax LaserComb from Lexington International LLC*
This device is one of only three treatments that are FDA-approved for hair growth. Dr. Rohrer says that "in a twenty-six-week, multicenter, placebo-controlled study with this device, 93% of subjects noticed an increase in hair count."

**3. Acne devices:** *Zeno MD from Tyrell and ClearTouch Lite from Radiancy*
Both devices thermally treat acne lesions and, according to Dr. Rohrer, Zeno achieved a 90% reduction in lesion counts in one to two days.

**4. Facial photorejuvenation:** *NuLase from NuLase International LLC and ClearTouch Lite from Radiancy*
Light-emitting diode devices are safe, relatively pain-free and can provide "subtle but real changes in the skin," says Dr. Rohrer.

**5. Facial toning:** *Facial toning device from Radiancy*
Dr. Rohrer claims the Radiancy device uses LHE (light and heat energy) technology and is capable of reducing age spots and wrinkles. However, the study he cited has not yet been published so we're more skeptical of this one.

# CAN A SKIN CREAM REALLY LIFT WRINKLES FROM THE INSIDE OUT?

*Erin wants to know:* I'm curious as to what you think about Garnier Nutritioniste Ultra-Lift. The advertising says, "It's skin care that actually lifts wrinkles from the inside out." How can the company say this?

The company can't say it, at least not anymore. According to the August 20, 2007 edition of *The Rose Sheet* (a cosmetics industry bulletin), L'Oreal, which owns Garnier, has been asked to modify or discontinue certain claims for Nutritioniste Ultra-Lift and Skin Renew products by the NAD (National Advertising Division). Here's a quick recap of the issues with three of L'Oreal's claims:

**1** **"...it actually lifts wrinkles from the inside out"**
What the NAD says: *"It is well established that topical creams do not absorb deep inside the skin in the same manner as cosmetic fillers such as collagen injections."* In other words, this lotion works from the outside in, not the other way around!

**2** **"...in three weeks wrinkles are visibly lifted and skin is noticeably firmer"**
What the NAD says: *In L'Oreal's clinical study, the questions "related to skin firmness refer to skin feeling firmer, not being noticeably firmer, as is explicitly stated in one of the challenged claims."*

**3** **Ultra-Lift "refuels cells within skin's deepest surface layers"**
What the NAD says: *L'Oreal's nine-week study showed Ultra-Lift's effect on fine lines, shallow wrinkles, tactile roughness and skin laxity. This is inadequate "particularly with regard to hydration—despite the presence of moisture-locking ingredients Omega 3 and 6."*

To be fair, we should point out that the NAD is not saying this product doesn't work at all. For example, the NAD did recognize that "scientific articles presented by the advertiser provide a reasonable basis for its ingredient claims in terms of accelerated cell proliferation and upped collagen production." It's just that L'Oreal didn't have adequate support for all the claims that it was making and so it has been asked to tone down its advertising.

## THE BOTTOM LINE

Ultra-Lift may make your skin feel better, but it's not going to actually get rid of your wrinkles.

# FIVE FASCINATING FACTS ABOUT MAX FACTOR COSMETICS

*Connie wants to win:* *Can you please settle a bet? My friend is trying to convince me that the Max Factor cosmetics line is really named after a guy named Max Factor. Sounds like an urban legend to me. I'm guessing it's really a marketing name like "Maximum Coverage Factor" or something like that. Please answer quickly. I can win an iTunes gift card!*

You can also *lose* an iTunes gift card, Connie. I'm afraid your friend is right: Max Factor Cosmetics is actually named after the chemist who created the company: Max Faktor.

Max is quite famous among us cosmetics chemists as one of the early pioneers of modern makeup. Here are few fun historical facts.

## FAKTOR TO FACTOR

Born in Poland in 1877, by the age of twenty Max was selling handmade rouges, fragrances and wigs. In 1902 he came to the United States where he changed his name from "Faktor" to "Factor," and by 1904 he was selling lotions and hair care products at the St. Louis World's Fair.

## SHOOT FOR THE STARS

In 1914 he created the first line of greasepaint products designed for motion picture stars. In just a few short decades, Jean Harlow, Claudette Colbert, Bette Davis and virtually all the major movie actresses were regular customers of the Max Factor beauty salon, located near Hollywood Boulevard.

## HE MADE UP MAKEUP

In the 1920s he developed a new line of color cosmetics for use in the new field of color motion pictures. In fact, he is credited with coining the word *makeup*.

## MAX AND OSCAR

In 1928 he was awarded a special technology Oscar from the Academy of Motion Picture Arts and Sciences for his makeup inventions. (Imagine that—a cosmetics chemist winning an Academy Award!)

## SELLING LIKE HOTCAKES

In the 1930s, Max Factor developed the first powder makeup in solid form, also known as pancake makeup, for film stars. When he made it available to the general public, pancake makeup became one of the biggest-selling products in the history of the cosmetics industry.

# HOW SALON BRANDS GET AWAY WITH LYING TO YOU

*Sally the salon operator writes:* I just noticed that the first ingredient listed in the Pureology shampoos and conditioners is now water. It's crazy how L'Oreal buys the brand and the first thing they do is "water down" the product (but not the price). My clients loved that there was no water in the products because they are so concentrated. What's the story?

The old Pureology shampoos and conditioners are good, although expensive, products. But just because the first ingredient is a botanical blend instead of water doesn't mean the products are more concentrated. And it certainly doesn't mean the products don't contain any water!

### SMALL COMPANIES CAN BE SNEAKY

What it really means is that Pureology was a small, independent salon company, and they chose not to follow the cosmetics labeling laws strictly. Many small companies use this trick of listing extracts first, thus making it look like they don't have any water. Don't fall for it! It's one of the oldest tricks in this industry and it's misleading and unfair. The formula is still mostly water!

Unfortunately, the Federal Trade Commission (FTC) and other agencies that fight this kind of consumer fraud are too busy with more serious issues and don't have time to chase after small companies that are tricking consumers with these kinds of labeling shenanigans.

### BIGGER COMPANIES FOLLOW THE LAW

Since L'Oreal is a much bigger company, it tends to play by the rules that all the big companies are held to. In the end, this is better for the consumer because you're getting more truth. Instead of being upset with L'Oreal, you should be thankful that it's labeling the products honestly.

And by the way, since L'Oreal has a much larger research staff than Pureology, any formula changes it makes are probably for the better!

# ARE MORE EXPENSIVE PRODUCTS WORTH THE PRICE?

*Grace wants to know:* Is it the quality really worth the increased price to pay for nondrugstore brands of cosmetics, skin care and hair care products?

This is one of the most common questions asked of the Beauty Brains. It warms our hearts because within the question is a kernel of skepticism that every beauty product consumer should harbor. It's also a thing that cosmetics marketers and manufacturers don't want you to have. It makes their jobs that much tougher!

To answer your question, we first have to make sure we're both on the same page. We assume that you are wondering whether the more expensive nondrugstore brands (like those found in salons, department stores and spas) perform better, are better for you or are otherwise superior to drugstore products.

## MORE EXPENSIVE PRODUCTS DO NOT WORK BETTER

From a performance standpoint, no, there is no reason to pay for higher-priced products. There have been numerous studies that demonstrate that expensive beauty products do not perform better than drugstore brands. In 2006, *Consumer Reports* reviewed face creams and found no correlation between how much they cost and how well they worked. Similar results were found by the BBC, which broadcast a documentary about anti-aging creams in 2007, and by a 2008 French consumer watchdog group study. The conclusion of all the most thorough work so far is simple:

*More expensive does not equal better working.*

And this makes sense if you consider the following.

## THE INGREDIENTS AREN'T DIFFERENT

In the United States, cosmetics and personal care products are all made from ingredients listed in the INCI (*International Nomenclature of Cosmetic Ingredients Dictionary*). For the most part, any company can create formulas that work nearly as well as any other company. The cetearyl alcohol found in the expensive La Prairie skin products is no different than the cetearyl alcohol found in Olay.

## THE SAME COMPANY MAKES DIFFERENT-PRICED PRODUCTS

Another reason to avoid paying for higher-priced products is because they are often made by companies that offer similar products for a much lower price. In the cosmetics industry, big corporations like Procter & Gamble and Unilever sell numerous brands at different price points. For example, P&G makes hair care products under the brand Pantene, but they also make Herbal Essences and Head & Shoulders. These products frequently use the same technologies but have much different costs. The cost differences are not related to how well the formula performs, but rather to the marketing and advertising.

## MASS MARKET PRODUCTS ARE OFTEN BETTER TESTED

The final reason that it is not worth paying for more expensive brands is that they are often made by smaller companies that do not have large research and development staffs. They don't put nearly as much money into developing and testing the best possible products. In fact, the product development work is often done by a contract manufacturer and not by the cosmetics company itself. Products from big companies that sell in drugstores are much more thoroughly tested and perform better overall.

## WHEN YOU SHOULD PAY MORE

So, if you are concerned about performance, then you should not buy the highest-priced cosmetics and personal care products. However, beauty products are not just about performance. Most people like the experience that goes along with using a beauty product. If this is your concern, then it may be worth it to you to spend more for your products. Factors like fragrance, packaging and brand name can all influence how happy you are with your purchase. If you can't feel good about yourself by having a Suave shampoo bottle in your shower, spending the extra money for Paul Mitchell might be worth it to you. Just don't expect it to work better…it probably won't.

## THE BOTTOM LINE

As we've said many times, if you like a product and you can afford it, buy it. But if you're buying a product because of hype you hear from the company that sells it, you're being fooled. Save your money and buy something less expensive!

# WHY DOES THE BEAUTY INDUSTRY GET AWAY WITH MAKING BOGUS CLAIMS?

*Maryellen wonders: Why is the beauty industry allowed to claim what they claim, as most of it is really bogus? How did this develop over time?*

We've written extensively about how cosmetics companies trick you but, to be fair, very little of what they specifically claim is bogus. There are relatively few occasions when companies tell out-and-out lies. When they do, they get fined or closed down by the government. So, where does the impression come from that the beauty industry marketers lie, even when they don't? Simple—marketing people are creative wordsmiths who know how to mislead you without actually lying.

## THEY DON'T EXACTLY LIE

If you look closely at advertisements, you'll find the things they claim are not lies.

For example, look at the Boots product claims in its No7 Protect & Perfect Beauty Serum.

(1) *Anti-Aging is getting Intense…No7 Protect & Perfect Intense Beauty Serum has been tested like no other cosmetic anti-aging product in an independent 12 month trial. (2) The findings clearly show that it has genuine, long-term anti-aging benefits. (3) 70% of the volunteers using the product showed a marked improvement in the appearance of photoaged skin after 12 months of use. (4) This proven anti-aging formula contains retinyl palmitate, antioxidants, firming peptides and alfalfa extract to reduce the appearance of deep lines and wrinkles by up to 50% in just 4 weeks, the longer you use it the better it works.*

Claim (1) is very likely true. Of course, every product is tested like no other!

It's difficult to say whether claim (2) is bogus because company spokespeople do not define "anti-aging benefits" nor how long "long term" is. Keeping things vague allows them to build up expectations in your mind without actually lying.

Claim (3) is likely true. But notice they do not explain what they mean by "marked improvement." Was this what the people who used the product thought, or was it the people running the test or someone else? It matters.

Claim (4) is absolutely true, since the product does contain all those things. What is not clear is what they mean by "proven anti-aging formula." Also, they say the product contains these things to "reduce the *appearance* of wrinkles" not to actually "reduce wrinkles." The word *appearance* is critical to keeping the statement true.

Perhaps all these claims together give you the impression that the product should work better than it does, but there are no specific lies.

In the U.S., television stations are held accountable for everything they broadcast and it is illegal for them to air false advertising. They can be fined or eventually shut down by the Federal Trade Commission (FTC). So the TV people strictly require that statements made in every commercial be backed up by some kind of evidence.

## SOMETIMES THEY DO GET IN TROUBLE

While beauty companies do have great copywriters, sometimes they get in trouble. Recently, L'Oreal was cited for using an actress with false eyelashes to promote mascara. P&G was forced to withdraw an ad for Olay because the ad's creators airbrushed the image of the model to make her look better.

## STORIES SELL PRODUCTS BETTER THAN PERFORMANCE

Most beauty products work about the same. Shampoos may smell different or feel a little different, but the vast majority of people would not notice differences if they tested these products on a blinded basis. For this reason, beauty companies have had to come up with better and better stories to make themselves stand out. When you can't stand out based on performance, you can always tell a better story.

## PEOPLE WANT TO BE DECEIVED

The thing is that people seem to want to be deceived. They want to believe that hair can be restored or that wrinkles can be made to vanish. They want to believe that they are not wasting money when they spend $300 on a face cream. The cosmetics industry is just giving people what they want. Unfortunately, most of the significant problems related to beauty have not been adequately solved by cosmetics scientists. We continue to look for better solutions, but they are slow to develop.

## THE BOTTOM LINE

While it is frustrating, and it might seem as if the cosmetics industry does nothing but lie, there are few instances of outright lying going on. For the most part, beauty companies tell the truth, but they do it in such a way that you are left with the impression that their products work better than they actually do. It is up to consumers to pay attention to what they read and think about claims they hear. If it sounds too good to be true, it probably is.

# WHAT DOES HYPOALLERGENIC MEAN?

*Kathy's query:* I was wondering what the most hypoallergenic makeup out there is. I have heard that all makeup is hypoallergenic, but I can't believe this is true. There are many brands that I cannot even look at, let alone use, without breaking out.

There is no universal standard for what constitutes hypoallergenic. Since each company is free to create its own guidelines, there's no way to tell which brand is the "most" hypoallergenic.

## HYPE-O-ALLERGENIC

According to the FDA,

hypoallergenic cosmetics are products that manufacturers claim produce fewer allergic reactions than other cosmetic products. Consumers with hypersensitive skin, and even those with "normal" skin, may be led to believe that these products will be gentler to their skin than nonhypoallergenic cosmetics.

There are no federal standards or guidelines that govern the use of the term *hypoallergenic*. The term means whatever a particular company wants it to mean. Manufacturers of cosmetics labeled as *hypoallergenic* are not required to submit substantiation of their hypoallergenicity claims to the FDA.

Furthermore, the FDA cautions that the word *hypoallergenic* has advertising value but "Dermatologists say it has very little meaning."

## THE BOTTOM LINE

Sadly, you can't necessarily tell if a product will be good for your skin by whether or not it claims to be hypoallergenic. Instead, look for brands that have a good reputation and that avoid ingredients like fragrance that are known irritants. And once you find a product that works for you, stick with it.

# WHAT'S THE DIFFERENCE BETWEEN COSMETICS AND DRUGS?

*Renée writes:* Why are antiperspirants and antidandruff products considered drugs, not cosmetics?

Legally speaking, a product is determined to be a cosmetic or a drug based on its intended use.

## LEGAL DEFINITIONS

U.S. law defines cosmetics as "articles intended to be rubbed, poured, sprinkled, or sprayed on, introduced into, or otherwise applied to the human body…for cleansing, beautifying, promoting attractiveness, or altering the appearance."

Drugs, on the other hand, are "articles intended for use in the diagnosis, cure, mitigation, treatment, or prevention of disease" and "articles (other than food) intended to affect the structure or any function of the body of man or other animals."

## DOUBLE DUTY

Some products (like the ones you asked about) provide both a cosmetic and a drug benefit. Antiperspirants make you smell better and antidandruff shampoos clean your hair; these are both cosmetic functions. But they also make drug claims: Antiperspirants stop you from sweating and antidandruff shampoos stop your scalp from flaking. These are physiological processes and any product that treats such conditions is automatically considered to be a drug. Other cosmetics that are classified as drugs include anticavity toothpastes and certain anti-itch lotions.

## THE BOTTOM LINE

You should also know that cosmetics that are classified as drugs have to comply with additional regulations related to good manufacturing processes, more rigorous stability testing and special labeling on the package.

# 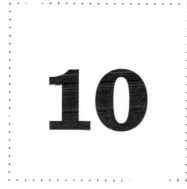 10 COSMETIC CONCERNS AND PERILOUS PRODUCTS

On the one hand, you have the cosmetics companies telling you how their products will miraculously enhance your beauty. On the other hand, you're told that those same products are full of chemicals that will penetrate your skin and poison you. In this chapter we'll explain whether or not you should be picky about ingredients like parabens or nanoparticles and we'll explain the surprising reason why sometimes it's actually OK to have toxins in your beauty products. We'll also give you the scoop on bizarre ingredients like foreskin, urine and spermicide. In this chapter you'll even learn how to tell if your cosmetics have gone bad and which products to avoid when you're pregnant.

# ARE YOUR COSMETICS POISONING YOU?

*Tracy is troubled:* I saw this newspaper headline that says women absorb up to five pounds of damaging chemicals a year from their beauty products. I'm amazed, astonished and perplexed. Can it be true?

We figured the article you mentioned was just a typical "scare" piece designed to spook us into fearing chemicals, but the article actually provides a reference to its headline and quotes from a biochemist. So we were intrigued. Are we really absorbing pounds of chemicals through our skin? We had to see the proof. The actual quote from the article is "The average woman absorbs 4 lbs, 6 oz of chemicals from toiletries and makeup every year, the industry magazine *In-Cosmetics* recently reported."

## NEWSWORTHY SOURCES

Here's where it gets interesting. First of all, *In-Cosmetics* is not a peer-reviewed scientific journal; it's a magazine published in conjunction with an annual trade show where companies that sell ingredients in cosmetics go to show off their newest products. Secondly, the quote appeared in an article titled "Trends in natural and organic cosmetics and toiletries."

It turns out that the notion that women absorb five pounds of chemicals a year from cosmetics comes from a scientist who runs a natural-products company called Spiezia Organics. According to Dr. Mariano Spiezia and his wife, Loredana, "Everything we need to be fulfilled and healthy is provided by nature. Today's research suggests that the human body will absorb most of what is applied to the skin, meaning that up to 2 kg (5 pounds) of chemicals a year from toiletries and skincare preparations."

There is no other reference provided. No studies are cited. Dr. Spiezia makes this assertion without making it clear what data he is basing it on. Without a clear foundation, this is junk science. The reporter just quotes it as fact. It is not fact. It is nonsense. It is the kind of junk science that some natural or organic companies try to dupe you into believing so you won't feel bad about spending your hard-earned money on their overpriced products.

## DO YOU ABSORB FIVE POUNDS OF COSMETICS CHEMICALS THROUGH YOUR SKIN EACH YEAR?

Based on our knowledge of the barrier properties of skin, this claim seems ridiculous. It suggests that skin is a sponge that absorbs any chemical it's exposed to. In fact, skin is just the opposite. It is actually a barrier that prevents chemicals from getting inside your body.

It's not a perfect barrier because some compounds do pass through the skin, like some sunscreens (e.g., benzophenone-3) and drugs like nicotine. So scientists are concerned about chemicals on the skin. But safety studies are conducted on chemicals all the time and the vast majority don't behave that way.

For the most part, the raw materials in cosmetics do not penetrate the skin so deeply that they are absorbed into the bloodstream. They are typically absorbed into only the top layer of skin (the stratum corneum) and are naturally removed over time through exfoliation.

## THE BOTTOM LINE

No, your cosmetics are not poisoning you. Chemicals can be absorbed through your skin, but that is true of only a small number of them and these have not been shown to cause problems. You certainly don't absorb five pounds of chemicals through your skin each year. The important thing to remember when you hear claims like this in the media is to check the source. Occasionally, it's backed up by science, but usually it is propaganda disseminated by a biased source. Proof is found in scientific studies, not in the opinions of natural-product selling "experts."

# SHOULD YOU WORRY ABOUT URINE IN YOUR MAKEUP?

*Meagan muses:* I've got a question about diazolidinyl urea. I see it on labels for lotions and cleansers all the time. Doesn't urea come from urine? That seems disgusting! What's the story?

Let's start by explaining that "diazolidinyl urea" is a preservative and it's used in many cosmetics to keep microscopic bugs from spoiling the products you bought with your hard-earned money. It so happens that urea is one of the compounds used to make this ingredient. In addition, urea is also used in some creams and lotions as a moisturizer. So urea is used in cosmetics, but does urea really come from urine? Well, urine *does* contain urea. That's because urea excretion is just one of the ways your body gets rid of the excess nitrogen waste material that it generates. Different animals process this waste in different ways: Aquatic organisms excrete it in the form of ammonia. Reptiles and birds excrete it in the form of uric acid. And we humans excrete it in the form of urea.

## DOES UREA COME FROM URINE?

Fret not: The source of the urea used to make ingredients in cosmetics is not someone's bladder. Industrial urea is made synthetically in large chemical reactors, which are rarely, if ever, peed into. As a matter of fact, urea was the *first* organic chemical ever to be synthesized from inorganic raw materials. Back in 1828 chemist Friedrich Woehler combined potassium cyanate with ammonium sulfate to create urea!

So, in summary, the basic message is that we should all get down on our knees right now and thank Dr. Woehler for inventing urea so we don't have to worry about whether or not some stranger had to pee in our Clinique lotion in order to stop bacteria from growing in it.

Or something like that.

## THE BOTTOM LINE

Urea is found in cosmetics, but it does not come from urine.

# THE PERILS OF PARABENS

*Shelly says:* Everyone is afraid of parabens! The product line that I use (Bioelements) lists methylparaben and propylparaben as the last ingredients, and I know that they are preservatives. But how do I know if they're safe when everyone is saying "Parabens = Bad!"

Parabens are preservatives used in nearly every kind of cosmetic. They are put in formulas in small amounts to prevent the growth of disease-causing microbes. Without preservatives, cosmetics would be much more dangerous to use. Parabens have been used in cosmetics for at least twenty years and are quite effective at killing microbes.

It's not surprising that parabens raise so many questions. Stories about these ingredients and the perils of using products that contain them are found everywhere on the Net. A quick Google search of parabens and cancer results in over 300,000 hits! Some sites decry the evils of parabens while others state a much different, less alarming position. So whom should you believe?

The FDA believes that, at present, there is no reason for consumers to be concerned about the use of cosmetics containing parabens. But FDA officials are still looking at the data.

## WHY DO PEOPLE THINK PARABENS ARE BAD?

So, where did the furor about parabens and cancer come from? In 2004, Dr. Philippa Darbre at the University of Reading published a study in the *Journal of Applied Toxicology* that said her group tested twenty different human breast tumors and found parabens in all of them. Neither she nor anyone else could explain how they got there or why they were there.

They also couldn't say whether normal tissue had parabens. This raised the possibility that the parabens could have something to do with the cancer, but no one could explain what was going on. And since then, no one has come up with a conclusive explanation. This doesn't mean parabens have anything to do with cancer. We just can't say that they don't.

## SO WHAT DO WE THINK?

Here at the Beauty Brains, we have to side with the majority of the scientific research. Namely, at the moment there's no significant reason to be concerned. The notion that parabens are a major cause of breast cancer is just not true! It's possible that they might play a role in breast cancer, but there is no conclusive evidence that supports this idea. No matter how bad parabens are, microbes are much worse.

Many cosmetics industry suppliers are offering alternatives to parabens. Privately, these companies acknowledge that parabens are more effective than the alternatives. They also do not believe there are any real safety issues, but it is an opportunity to create new products so they are taking it.

Unfortunately, every other effective preservative such as DMDM hydantoin (a formaldehyde-releasing ingredient) or kathon (a synthetic) have potential safety issues. And suggested alternatives like grapefruit seed extract, phenoxyethanol, potassium sorbate, sorbic acid, tocopherol (vitamin E), vitamin A (retinyl), vitamin C (ascorbic acid) don't really work too well. The available preservatives aren't perfect, but they are the best there is at this time. And they are certainly better than using nothing. The bacteria, yeast and mold that parabens prevent really could kill you!

## THE BOTTOM LINE

Preservative alarmists may have a point and the industry is constantly on the lookout for new, effective ingredients. They just haven't found any. But the risk posed from these ingredients is so small that it's not worth worrying about. There are more critical things you can do to keep from getting cancer, like not smoking, avoiding excessive sun exposure, exercising regularly and eating a well-balanced, low-fat diet. Don't waste your energy fretting about the preservatives in your cosmetics.

# WHY ARE THERE DIFFERENT KINDS OF PARABENS IN PRODUCTS?

*Natalie asks: I know that parabens are preservatives, but why are products formulated with multiple variations of them? I have products with methylparaben, ethylparaben, propylparaben, butylparaben (or a combination) in them. Do they have different functions?*

Parabens seem to have developed a scary reputation, which is unfortunate because they are amazing compounds that make disease-free cosmetics and food possible. As we discussed above, they have a long history of safe use and there is scant evidence that they are causing any health problems.

You are correct that they are common preservatives and you'll find them in creams, lotions, color cosmetics and almost any other personal care product. They are actually used extensively in food, too. They are some of the most safe and effective compounds cosmetics chemists can use.

Compounds like methylparaben and ethylparaben are classified as parabens because they have the same basic structure (parahydroxybenzoic acid) with only slight modifications. Methylparaben is the simplest, followed by ethyl-, propyl- and butyl-. All effectively kill bacteria and fungi that can spoil cosmetics and spread disease.

There are two primary reasons that companies use multiple versions of parabens in formulas.

## 1 Different parabens, different effectiveness

Since each paraben is chemically different, it kills microbes to a different degree. Methylparaben is probably the most effective, but there are some bacteria that ethylparaben works better on. Similarly, propylparaben and butylparaben are more effective on certain types of microbes. When formulators include all the different parabens, they are reducing the chances that contamination will ever be a problem.

## 2 Oil and water compatibility

The chemical differences in parabens also mean that they have different compatibilities with water and oil. Methylparaben mixes well with water but not as well with oil. Butylparaben doesn't combine with water at all. Creams and lotions are made up of both oil and water, so different preservatives have to be used for each phase. Multiple preservatives ensure that the entire formula is preserved.

## THE BOTTOM LINE

Multiple types of parabens are used in formulas to ensure that your personal care and cosmetics products are as free as possible from disease-causing microbes. They make products safe from spoilage and help prevent the spread of disease.

# SHOULD YOU BE WORRIED ABOUT SPERMICIDE IN YOUR SPA CREAM?

*Teresa has trepidations:* I was shopping for high-end spa products and noticed that their exfoliant cream contains nonoxynol-9, a famously debated spermicide ingredient! I'm assuming it's not there to keep my freshly smoothed skin from becoming pregnant. So why is it in my cream and is there any downside to using it?

Nonoxynol-9 (or N-9) is in your spa cream to help dissolve the oil-soluble ingredients in the cream base. That's because it's a surfactant (which is short for surface active agent), which is just a fancy way of saying it's a type of detergent. The cool thing is that N-9 is a nonionic surfactant, which is a special type that doesn't create a lot of lather. Otherwise, the spa cream would get all foamy when you rub it into your skin.

## DETERGENTS CAN BE SPERMICIDAL

It just so happens that N-9's ability to dissolve oil into water has a very important side effect—it can also dissolve the acrosomal membranes of sperm, which stops the little guys from swimming. That's why it's used in many spermicidal creams, jellies, foams, gels, films and suppositories. So N-9 serves double duty: shy spa-cream emulsifier by day; sultry sperm killer by night.

## THE BOTTOM LINE

Nonoxynol-9 is found in both skin creams and spermicides, but it's perfectly safe for your face.

# MYTHS ABOUT MINERAL OIL

We often see the advice that people should avoid mineral oil at all costs. This idea is propagated by numerous "natural" companies. Well, this advice is just bogus and is not based on any scientific studies. Mineral oil is a perfectly fine ingredient and has been used in cosmetics for over one hundred years.

Here are the top five myths that companies tell people to make them afraid of mineral oil.

**1** **Mineral oil is contaminated with carcinogens.** While it's true that some petroleum derivatives contain carcinogenic materials (such as some polycyclic aromatic compounds), the mineral oil that is used in the cosmetics and pharmaceutical industry is highly refined and purified. Its purity is even regulated by the U.S. FDA and other international regulatory agencies. There is absolutely no evidence that cosmetics-grade mineral oil causes cancer. And there has been plenty of testing done to ensure that fact. We could find no published reports in any of the dermatological or medical journals indicating a link between mineral oil and any forms of cancer.

**2** **Mineral oil dries the skin and causes premature aging.** Mineral oil works as a barrier between the skin and the air. It acts as an occlusive agent, which means that it prevents water from naturally leaving your body through your skin. It will not dry out your skin or cause premature aging. Quite the contrary. It acts as a moisturizer.

**3** **Mineral oil robs the skin of vitamins.** Since many vitamins are oil-based, people assume that mineral oil will pull vitamins out of your skin. No legitimate scientific evidence makes this claim. Mineral oil has no effect on the vitamin levels in your skin.

**4** **Mineral oil prevents absorption of collagen from collagen moisturizers.** Collagen molecules in your skin lotions and moisturizers are too big to actually penetrate your skin. Therefore, mineral oil will have no effect on whether the collagen gets absorbed or not.

**5** **Mineral oil causes acne.** In some people, mineral oil can exacerbate acne problems. However, most people will not experience any problems.

So, if it is not for safety concerns, why would companies be telling you to avoid mineral oil? Here are a few reasons why:

**1** **They want you to buy from them, instead of the big manufacturers.** This is the primary explanation for mineral oil bashing. Little companies have to find a way to convince consumers to use their products instead of the less expensive name brands produced by large manufacturers. They can't possibly advertise as much as the big guys, so they need other ways to motivate consumers to choose their products.

And most people don't have the time or scientific background to question what they hear. They'll just believe a myth about mineral oil causing cancer and avoid it at all costs. The lack of skepticism in our country is extremely troubling to the Beauty Brains.

**2** **They need to have a reason why their products don't work as well.** The truth is that mineral oil is one of the best-functioning skin care ingredients available. Every cosmetics chemist who reads studies published in the *Journal of the Society of Cosmetic Chemists* knows it. Other oils work, too, but not as well as mineral oil.

When chemists are told that they need to create a formula without mineral oil to respond to a media scare story, they can't produce the best-functioning product out there because they have to compromise performance with less effective ingredients.

**3** **They think natural things are inherently good.** You find this notion throughout society, but especially in the areas of cosmetics. In the United States, some people automatically believe that something taken directly from nature is better than something that is human-made or synthetic. Of course, there is no evidence supporting this notion and plenty of evidence to show that it is wrong. Natural is not necessarily better! Snake venom is natural. Cyanide is natural. Uranium is natural. Natural can be both good and bad. Similarly, synthetic things can be both good and bad.

The thing that is most amusing is that mineral oil is itself "natural." It is pulled right out of Mother Earth and purified for use in your favorite cosmetics. There is no synthetic process involved, just simple distillation of naturally occurring oil.

**4** **They believe all the myths about mineral oil.** Despite the fact that there are some companies that are just trying to scare and lie to you, there are some people who honestly believe everything they've read about the evils of mineral oil. And who could blame them? We all lead busy lives and when you hear bits of information that sound plausible, you don't have time to read the supporting research. Consequently, manufacturers might believe they've found a much better product when they really haven't. People want to believe they can solve other people's problems. Even if their solution is based on a delusion.

# WHAT YOU SHOULD KNOW ABOUT PREGNANCY AND COSMETICS

*Fran speaks frankly:* *I've heard that you should avoid putting certain ingredients on your skin when you're pregnant. Are salicylic acid, self-tanners and sunscreens safe to use when you're expecting? Are there any other ingredients or skin care products pregnant women should avoid?*

Experts agree that you should limit unnecessary drug exposure when you're pregnant. Here's what we found out from two expert sources: the American Pregnancy Association and the American Academy of Dermatologists.

## FIVE FACTS ABOUT PREGNANCY AND SKIN CARE INGREDIENTS

**1** **Retin-A (Isotretinoin)** is a prescription acne medication that can cause cardiac problems in a fetus.

**2** **Minoxidil (aka Rogaine),** the over-the-counter hair restoration drug, is also known to contribute to birth defects.

**3** **Fluconazole** is a topical antifungal drug that can also be teratogenic (meaning, it causes birth defects).

**4** **Sunscreens and sunless tanners** appear to be fine. There have been no reports of babies born with problems related to the mother's use of sunscreens. In fact, since UV radiation may cause folic acid deficiency, which can lead to neural tube defects like spina bifida, sunscreens could actually help!

**5** **Salicylic acid facial products** are apparently low risk as well. But muscle creams containing a related compound (methyl salicylate) can be dangerous if overused, even if you're not pregnant.

## THE BOTTOM LINE

You should avoid certain medications and products when you're pregnant, and be sure to check with your doctor to make sure you're doing everything right for you and your baby's health.

# FIVE WAYS BEAUTY PRODUCTS CAN GO BAD

**Cayley is quizzical:** *Do beauty products have expiration dates hidden on the package? Whenever I see a great deal for an expensive beauty product on eBay or at a discount store like Marshalls, I wonder if the product has expired and is no longer as effective.*

There's no way to tell if a cosmetic has expired just by looking at the package, but we can tell you what to look for when products go bad.

**1 Change in odor**
Fragrances are made of dozens of different ingredients that can react with the rest of the product. It's not surprising, then, that the fragrance is often the first thing to go bad. A little fragrance fading is totally normal, but if you detect a sour or rancid odor, it may be a sign that something is seriously wrong.

**2 Color shifting**
The color of the product is very sensitive to light, so it's not unusual for cosmetics in clear packaging to experience a shift in shade. Slight color changes don't necessarily mean there's anything functionally wrong with the product, but you certainly don't want your red lipstick to become too orangey.

**3 Change in texture**
Changes in the consistency of a product may be subtle but significant. For example, if your skin lotion looks exceptionally thick or thin, or if it appears too grainy, this may be an early indicator of emulsion instability. This means the oil- and water-soluble chemicals are separating. Not good!

**4 Microbial contamination**
If you see any black spots or fuzzy growth in your product, it could be contaminated with bacteria or fungus. Get rid of it immediately or you may be at risk for infection! And by the way, you should never dilute a product with water just so you can get the last little bit out of the bottle. Adding water can dilute the preservative system, which can allow potentially dangerous bugs to grow.

**5 Physical separation**
If the product has separated into two layers, it has gone bad. You can't always fix it by just remixing it. This is particularly true of cosmetics that have active ingredients, like sunscreens and dandruff shampoos. Once the active drug ingredient has separated from the rest of the formula, it may not work properly anymore.

## DO COSMETICS HAVE EXPIRATION DATES?

In the United States, cosmetic products are not required to have expiration dates. That's not really a bad thing because it's difficult, if not impossible, to predict the exact shelf life of any given cosmetic products. (European products, on the other hand, must be stamped with a Period After Opening date.) The shelf life of any given product depends, at least in part, on how it's stored. Products can be stable for several years if they're kept away from light and heat, the two biggest enemies of cosmetics. But that same product can start to show fragrance degradation and color shift in a few weeks if exposed to sunlight and/or high temperatures.

The exceptions are over-the-counter drugs like dandruff shampoos, antiperspirants, fluoride toothpastes and acne products. The activity of drug ingredients in these products can be measured over time to estimate an expiration date. But it doesn't work that way for nondrug products, and for the vast majority of cosmetic products it's a guessing game.

## THE BOTTOM LINE

There's no way to tell just from looking at the package if the product is still good or not. But if you're really desperate there *is* one thing you might try: Look for the "secret" code that is the manufacturer's lot number. If you're shopping on eBay and you see a product that you like, you can email eBay and ask the seller if she can tell you the lot number on the package. Then you could contact the maker of the product and ask when it was made. That doesn't guarantee that the product is good, but at least you can get an idea of its age before you spend a lot of money on it.

# IS RADIATION FROM CELL PHONES AND COMPUTERS BAD FOR YOUR SKIN?

*Billie smells a bogus claim:* I read about a Clarins product called Expertise 3P Mist, which supposedly protects your skin from the electromagnetic effects of cell phones and computers. Is this something that we should be concerned about? Seems like it's dressed-up toner. Would love your insight.

This has got to be one of the most ridiculous new products we've heard about in a long time.

This product does appear to be a typical toner. While we couldn't find a complete ingredients list, we were amused to read about its "Magnetic Defense Complex with Thermus Chermophilus and Rhodiola Rosea, two powerful plant extracts which reinforce the skin's natural barrier and provide biological protection against electromagnetic waves." Please! This can't possibly work. To block electromagnetic fields, you would need some kind of metal or insulator. This is just ridiculous.

## THE BOTTOM LINE

Even if these ingredients *did* absorb electromagnetic radiation, you'd have to smear them *all* over your body before they would protect you. And finally, even if these ingredients *did* work and even if you *did* apply the product all over your body, there is absolutely no demonstrated negative effect on skin due to the electromagnetic fields created by cell phones or computers. We say save your money and don't sweat the "scary" electromagnetic fields.

# IS FORESKIN GOOD FOR YOUR FACE?

**Christie is curious:** *There is a product called TNS Recovery Complex by Skin Medica that is made from (how can I say this tastefully?) a discarded piece of skin that some parents opt to have removed from their newborn baby boys before they leave the hospital. My dermatologist recommends and sells it. It has also been talked about enthusiastically on Oprah. Does this product really live up to the hype as an anti-aging, antiwrinkle cream? It is very expensive!*

According to the Skin Medica website, TNS contains an ingredient called Nouricel-MD, which is the company's trade name for a combination of natural growth factors, matrix proteins and soluble collagen. Natural growth factors are a new category of compounds that act as chemical messengers to turn on and off a variety of cellular activities.

## DO NATURAL GROWTH FACTORS WORK?

Theoretically, these compounds could have anti-aging properties when used in cosmetics. However, although products like TNS do contain growth factors, it looks as if this technology is still in the experimental stages. According to Dr. Patricia Farris of the American Academy of Dermatologists, "A multi-center double-blinded clinical study is currently underway to assess the anti-aging effects of human growth factors, and I expect that we'll be hearing a lot about their potential in medical applications in the coming years." Until we see study results to the contrary, we assume this product is more marketing hype than scientific breakthrough.

## SHOW ME THE FORESKIN

But where did the notion that TNS contains foreskin come from? As the AAD article points out, growth factors can be extracted from plants, cultured epidermal cells, placental cells and human foreskins. Aha! Since growth factors *can* be derived from foreskin (as well as other sources) and since Skin Medica uses growth factors in its TNS product, you can see how someone could jump to the conclusion that TNS contains actual human foreskin.

In fact, according to Skin Medica, its Nouricel-MD ingredient was developed by a San Diego-based biotechnology company that patented a process for growing cell banks. So until Skin Medica announces that its secret ingredient is really based on infant penile sheaths, our guess is that this is just another internet rumor.

## THE BOTTOM LINE

The cells found in human foreskin may have anti-aging properties, but they're not yet found in any cosmetics.

# WILL COVERING YOUR BODY WITH ANTIPERSPIRANT SUFFOCATE YOU?

*Jessica is perspicacious about perspiration:* Is there any danger in applying antiperspirant on large areas of the body? For example, on the back, hairline and so on?

It sounds like you might have a case of hyperhydrosis, a condition that causes your sweat glands to kick into overdrive. So before we talk about antiperspirants, let's explain the source of sweat.

## WHERE DOES SWEAT COME FROM?

There are two types of sweat glands on your body: eccrine glands and apocrine glands. Eccrine glands are found all over your body but are most concentrated on the palms of hands, the soles of feet and the forehead. These glands produce sweat that is water and some salts and they are important in regulating body temperature. Sweat from eccrine glands doesn't cause body odor.

Apocrine glands are not as widespread. They are always associated with hair follicles so they show up wherever there is body hair, such as in your armpits and…uh…other areas. Apocrine glands produce a milky sweat that contains fatty materials. Bacteria that feed on these fatty materials create the unique smell of sweat.

## HOW DO ANTIPERSPIRANTS STOP SWEATING?

The active ingredients in antiperspirants are aluminum salts. Aluminum ions from these salts are absorbed by the cells that line the eccrine gland ducts. When water mixes with the salt, the cells swell up and form a plug that closes the gland, so more sweat can't get out. A typical antiperspirant can decrease your sweat by at least 20 percent. Extra-strength products, available by prescription, are even more effective.

## CAN YOU USE ANTIPERSPIRANT ALL OVER YOUR BODY?

This question reminds us of the story of the actress in the James Bond film *Goldfinger* who supposedly died from asphyxiation after being covered with gold paint. Fortunately, this story turns out to be an urban myth—your body doesn't "breathe" through your skin so you can't really suffocate. However, eccrine glands do help control body temperature, and if you blocked all your sweat glands, your body would be in danger of overheating.

We couldn't find any medical references that explained exactly how much antiperspirant poses a danger. The best we could come up with is this reference from Unilever (makers of Degree) warning that antiperspirants are "…really only designed for reducing underarm sweat and they should never be sprayed all over your body as you may overheat if too many sweat glands are blocked."

That seems like a reasonable caution to us but it's not a very satisfying answer if you're drenched in sweat.

## THE BOTTOM LINE

If hyperhydrosis is really a problem, we'd suggest checking with your doctor about using prescription-strength antiperspirants or even more drastic measures, like electrical treatments or Botox injections, that can temporarily stun the sweat glands. It's probably not a good idea to use antiperspirant on parts of your body other than your underarms.

# THREE REASONS WHY IT'S OK TO HAVE TOXINS IN COSMETICS

*Lin longs to learn:* I read on a medical website that ammonium hydroxide is a toxin and is found in many industrial products and cleaners such as flooring strippers, brick cleaners and cements. I've noticed it in several skin care products (like NeoStrata AHA gel) and I'm worried. Worst of all, they warn you not to get it on your skin or in your eyes. Why is this toxic chemical in cosmetics?

Consumers should be asking questions like this to find out if their cosmetics are safe. But, believe it or not, a lot of cosmetics (and food products!) contain ingredients that can be harmful at high concentrations. It's actually perfectly safe to use ingredients like these as long as they're formulated properly. Here are three reasons why it's OK to have a toxic chemical in cosmetics.

**1 It's present at low levels.**
The ingredient can be added to the formula at such a low level that it has no negative effect whatsoever. Some preservatives are irritating when applied directly to the skin. But when used at very low levels in a product, they are much more easily tolerated by most people.

**2 It's used up in a reaction.**
The ingredient can be used up or chemically reacted so it's not actually present in the finished product in a harmful form. Ammonium hydroxide is a good example of this type: It reacts with acidic materials in the formula and is neutralized to form a safe salt.

**3 It's not abused.**
The ingredient can be dangerous if abused, but is safe if used properly. For example, a hair relaxer is very dangerous if you swallow it or get it in your eyes. But when you use this toxic product properly, there's usually no problem. (Although some people do find relaxers irritating.)

## THE BOTTOM LINE

We're not saying that *all* toxic ingredients should be treated as safe; we're just saying that you shouldn't overreact to something you read on a website when the information is taken out of context. Ammonium hydroxide is not something you have to worry about in your skin lotion.

# ARE NATURAL PRODUCTS BETTER THAN PROCESSED?

*Shara wants to know:* I've heard about parasites in Baby's Bliss Gripe Water. What's the story?

The FDA has reported that the parasite cryptosporidium has, indeed, been found in this product. People who have given Mom Enterprises' Baby's Bliss Gripe Water to their infants now have the added benefit of knowing they may have given them a parasite, too. If you are one of those parents who have a bottle with code 26952V and an expiration date of October 2008, throw away or return the product immediately.

## HERBAL SUPPLEMENT OUTRAGE

Herbal supplement companies are not regulated, and the FDA does not have enough resources to test every supplement product put on the market, so you have no way of knowing whether the product is safe or not. Unlike food manufacturers, there is no law that requires independent testing of the products made and sold by herbal supplement manufacturers. These supplements can have real health effects and it's only through sheer luck that problems are discovered.

## THE NONSENSE OF NATURAL PRODUCTS

Mom Enterprises also sells a line of personal care products. We hope that the company doesn't rely on the "naturalness" of its raw materials and treats them to remove disease-causing parasites, bacteria and viruses. These are the kinds of things that preservatives are designed to kill. Yes, preservatives protect us from the evil things found in natural products.

Mom Enterprises' Baby's Bliss makes a diaper cream the company claims to be "100% natural." Their list of ingredients includes the following:

*caprylic/capric triglyceride, cetyl alcohol, zinc oxide, cetearyl olivate (and) sorbitan olivate, stearic acid, dimethicone, glycine, fragrance.*

You can't find dimethicone in nature. It's derived from sand, but you have to go through a lot of chemical processing to make it. This product isn't 100 percent natural. It's processed, and that's a good thing. Processed products are safer products!

## THE BOTTOM LINE

When you don't process and chemically alter natural things, you end up with *parasites* or bacteria or other disease-causing microbes. That's not something you want. And if you are in the United States and you're giving herbal supplements to your children, you're taking a huge risk! The products are unregulated and in the Beauty Brains' opinion, unsafe for children.

# WHAT IS VIOLET #2 AND WHAT DOES IT DO?

*Elizabeth asks:* What is violet #2 and why is it used in body washes?

Violet #2, as you can probably guess from the name, is a violet color used in cosmetics. But there's much more to the story than just that!

## COLORFUL CHEMISTRY

The correct name for violet #2 is actually "D&C violet #2." The *D&C* stands for "Drug and Cosmetics," which indicates the types of products this dye can be used in. Some colors are classified as FD&C, which means they can be used in food, drugs and cosmetics. Others are just D&C. You can also refer to it by its scientific name, which is hydroxy-1 ((methyl-4 phenyl)amino)-4 anthracenedione-9,10. You see why it's just called it violet #2!

Violet #2, not surprisingly, can be used to color products purple. But combinations of red and blue dyes actually do a better job of making purple. So why use violet #2? Because it has a secret superpower that makes it especially useful in products that are *not* colored purple.

## ANTI-YELLOW AGENT

If you remember your basic physics, color is made up of different wavelengths of light. And colors made of opposing wavelengths can cancel each other out. Violet is the "opposite" of yellow, so the two cancel each other out, leaving no color at all. (This is a bit of an oversimplification, but you get the idea.)

So what does all this have to do with body wash? Some ingredients used in body washes and shampoos (especially the detergents and the fragrance) can cause a slight yellow color, especially as the product ages over time. Cosmetics scientists add a teeny-tiny bit of violet #2 to the formula to keep the product from looking yellow. Typically, this is done in products that are meant to look colorless. So the violet isn't there to make purple; it's there to stop the evil yellow!

## THE BOTTOM LINE

Violet #2 is in your body wash to keep it from turning yellow. It's the only colorant ingredient that's used with the purpose of *not* being able to see it. Isn't science cool?

# WHY ARE COMPANIES ALLOWED TO USE NANOPARTICLES?

**Jan wonders:** *I choose not to use consumer products with nanoparticles. However, I would like to know why they are permitted to be in cosmetics and skin care products when there may be serious health issues.*

There are a variety of reasons that nanoparticles are allowed in personal care, including lack of proof of harm, lack of regulation by the FDA and lack of knowledge about their effects.

## WHAT ARE NANOPARTICLES?

Nanoparticles are tiny particles that are seven to ten times smaller than a grain of sand. In many fields of study, like medicine and electronics, nanoparticles promise to revolutionize technology. In cosmetics, they have been used most frequently in sunscreens to help create products that protect users from the sun, but remain clear. For these applications, nanoparticles of titanium dioxide and zinc oxide are used. They have also been used in anti-aging products to help deliver active ingredients to the lower levels of skin.

## WHY ARE PEOPLE WORRIED?

Concerns about nanoparticles began when it was shown that some of the most promising ones (such as carbon nanotubes and buckyballs) could be toxic to animal cells. Other research suggests that they have the potential to damage DNA. It seems that when some chemicals get to be small enough, they take on different chemical properties. If the results from these studies are true outside the laboratory, it could be problematic.

Perhaps the biggest reason for concern is that people fear the unknown, especially when it comes to new chemical technologies. There is a tendency for many people to assume that something is harmful until it is proven otherwise. Unfortunately, you can never prove that something is harmless. You can only show a low probability of harm.

## NO PROOF OF HARM

One reason nanoparticles continue to be used is that no one has shown them to be harmful. Nanoparticles were first introduced into cosmetics in the early 1990s and have been used ever since. While some lab studies raise concerns, there have not been any studies to show that nanoparticles are capable of penetrating the skin or otherwise getting into the body. The belief is that if they can't get in, then they can't cause harm. We'll see if that is still the belief in a few years.

## NO REGULATION

Another reason they are still allowed in consumer products is because there are no regulations specifically covering nanoparticles. The FDA is monitoring the use of these compounds, but until there is some demonstrated problem, the FDA is powerless to act. It should be noted that there are regulations related to sunscreens; however, they were written before it was possible to deliberately create nanoparticles, so they don't apply. If there is a study showing that nanoparticles are harmful, the FDA will act to regulate them, but not until that happens.

## THE BOTTOM LINE

While there is the potential for nanoparticles to cause health problems, there is no proof that they are harmful, so beauty product makers will continue to use them. If you worry about chemical exposure, then it makes sense for you to avoid using products containing nanoparticles until more extensive research is done. For now, we're convinced that science shows that nanoparticles do not penetrate skin and are safe for use. But, as with everything, we could easily change our minds if the data warrant it. Keep paying attention to this issue as more research is done.

# WHAT'S WRONG WITH SULFATES?

**Martha wonders:** *What is the truth about sulfates? Also, what is the difference between ammonium lauryl/laureth sulfates and sodium lauryl/laureth sulfates? And is one safer or better than the other?*

If you spend any time on the internet looking at beauty products or reading chain emails, you've probably heard about sodium lauryl sulfate (SLS) and undoubtedly, it was something negative. It is one of the most vilified ingredients still commonly used in personal care products. Chemical fear mongers say it irritates skin, builds up in your internal organs, causes hair loss and even causes cancer. But is any of this true?

## EFFECTS OF SLS

SLS is a good, inexpensive detergent, which is why it is used in a wide range of personal care products. It can be derived from coconut oil or from petroleum. It is true that SLS can be irritating. In fact, when cosmetics companies do irritation patch tests, SLS is used as the positive control because it irritates the skin of almost everyone when exposed for a long time. This is why you don't want to leave SLS-containing shampoos and body washes on your skin for too long. It is fine for short-term exposure (less than ten minutes) but it gets irritating the longer it's on.

The rest of the claims about SLS are not supported by any scientific studies. There is no proof that SLS builds up, causes hair loss or causes cancer. These are fabricated claims designed to scare you into buying more expensive products from companies that don't use SLS.

## SODIUM AND AMMONIUM

One thing that has always struck us as odd is that while sodium lauryl sulfate is constantly bashed, ammonium lauryl sulfate (ALS) is almost never mentioned. But when put into a formula, there is almost no difference between the two! They are both low-cost detergents that do an excellent job of cleaning and foaming. The part of the molecule that is responsible for all the functionality is the same—lauryl sulfate.

ALS and SLS are salts similar to table salt. If you think back on grade school science, you might recall that salt is sodium chloride. When you put it in water, salt dissolves and separates into sodium ions and chlorine ions. The same thing happens to ALS and SLS. When SLS is put into the water of a cosmetic formula, it separates into sodium ions and lauryl sulfate ions. ALS also separates into ions, except that it has an ammonium ion instead of a sodium ion. Neither the sodium nor the ammonium ions have a significant effect on the overall formula.

## LAURYL AND LAURETH

The difference between sodium lauryl sulfate and sodium laureth sulfate (SLES) molecules is some extra oxygen. Laureth sulfates contain oxygen while lauryl sulfates don't. This difference does have an effect on the performance. In general, laureth sulfates foam less, clean a little less and are less irritating. Basically, cosmetic formulators created a gentler product that doesn't clean quite as well.

## WHICH ONE IS SAFER?

From a practical standpoint, none of these sulfates are any more or less safe than the others. As used in personal care products today, they are all safe. Some people will find SLS and ALS more irritating than SLES or ammonium laureth sulfate (ALES). But irritation does not reflect a lack of safety. Something can irritate the skin and still be "safe."

## THE BOTTOM LINE

While there are some subtle chemical differences between sodium lauryl sulfate and ammonium lauryl sulfate, there is no difference in performance or irritation level. Laureth sulfates are slightly less irritating, but are also slightly less cleansing than lauryl sulfates. When used as directed, all these compounds have been demonstrated to be safe.

# USEFUL RESOURCES

The Beauty Brains hope that by reading our book, everyone will become a smarter consumer who makes informed decisions when purchasing beauty products.

While you can learn something new every day on the Beauty Brains blog, there are a number of other great resources for finding more beauty product information and advice.

## CONSUMER REPORTS

*(www.consumerreports.org/cro/health-fittness/beauty-personal-care)*
This is the online version of the magazine. It features information about a variety of beauty and personal care products, including researched reports on sunscreens, wrinkle creams, anti-aging products and more. It provides well-researched and unbiased information.

## THE COSMETICS COP

*(www.cosmeticscop.com)*
Paula Begoun started her career as makeup artist, moved to television as a beauty reporter and finally became the Cosmetics Cop, authoring several best-selling books about the beauty industry, such as *Don't Go to the Cosmetics Counter without Me* and *The Beauty Bible*. Her website and books feature reviews of thousands of cosmetics and personal care products. She does an excellent job of reviewing both the products and some of the science behind them.

## QUACK WATCH

*(http://quackwatch.com)*
While this site is primarily dedicated to health-related topics, it provides an excellent foundation for critical thinking and evaluation of the claims, demos and bunk

used to sell cosmetics and beauty products. You can find a number of articles about how to protect yourself from quackery all around you.

## U.S. FOOD AND DRUG ADMINISTRATION

*(www.cfsan.fda.gov/~dms/cos-toc.html)*
Contrary to what some sources claim, the FDA does provide regulatory guidelines for the cosmetics industry. At this website you can find information about a number of cosmetics issues, such as ingredient and product descriptions, labeling requirements, recall information and even a quiz to test how smart you are about cosmetics.

## PERSONAL CARE PRODUCTS COUNCIL—COSMETICS INFO

*(www.cosmeticsinfo.org)*
This website is run by the Cosmetics Industry Oversight Council, which is responsible for ensuring that cosmetics in the U.S. comply with accepted standards. It provides good scientific information, but it is not completely unbiased, since it's run by cosmetics manufacturers.

## AMERICAN ACADEMY OF DERMATOLOGY

*(www.aad.org)*
This site provides a wealth of free information regarding nearly every type of skin condition known. You can find advice for how to deal with acne, eczema, psoriasis and other common skin problems. It also gives great information for finding a dermatologist in your area.

## SOCIETY OF COSMETIC CHEMISTS

*(www.scconline.org/website/news/ask_the_expert.shtml)*
If you want to know more about cosmetics, try the SCC's Ask the Expert page. Simply fill out the form and send in your question. It will be answered by a member of the Society of Cosmetic Chemists.

## THE DEMON-HAUNTED WORLD—SCIENCE AS A CANDLE IN THE DARK
### *BY CARL SAGAN*

Sagan was a wonderful writer and this book was one of his best works. In it he explained how science can be used to understand the world better. Of particular interest to skeptical beauty aficionados is chapter 12, in which there is a "baloney detection kit" for determining if something is science or fiction.

# INGREDIENTS LISTS

Perhaps the most important skill you can cultivate to evaluate cosmetics is reading the ingredients list. In the cosmetics business, it's called an LOI or list of ingredients. Here is how you read it, what it means and where you can find more information.

In the United States, cosmetics manufacturers are compelled by the governing industry trade organization, known as the Personal Care Products Council (formerly the Cosmetic, Toiletry and Fragrance Association), to include a list of ingredients on their labels. They maintain a book known as the INCI (*International Nomenclature of Cosmetic Ingredients Dictionary*) with the names of nearly all the ingredients used in cosmetic products worldwide. It's quite a tome, and it makes for groovy bedtime reading.

## WHY THE LABELS?

The labels are required because the industry wants consumers to know exactly what chemicals they are putting on their bodies. This will allow you to make choices as to which chemicals you want to be exposed to.

Of course, this presumes that you know what any of the chemicals are, which for most consumers is not the case. Fortunately, with the internet you can simply look up chemical names using a search engine to get more information about the compounds. Be careful however: There are plenty of sites loaded with misinformation about perfectly safe chemicals. Compounds like propylene glycol, mineral oil and sodium lauryl sulfate have been slandered by biased sources all over the internet. Read all things on the internet with a skeptical eye. We reject gurus and encourage everyone to become his or her own expert.

## WHAT DO THE LABELS MEAN?

When properly written, the labels can provide you with a lot of useful information. In the United States, any chemicals above 1 percent by weight in the formula are required to be listed in order of concentration. Below 1 percent, they can be listed in any order. Typically, preservatives, fragrances and colors are listed at the end. As an example, let's look at the list of ingredients in a skin moisturizer:

water, glycerin, cetearyl alcohol, petrolatum, mineral oil, ceteareth 20, dimethicone, glyceryl dilaurate, erythrulose, persea gratissima fruit extract (avocado), avena sativa meal extract (oat), simmondsia chinensis seed extract (jojoba), calendula officinalis flower extract, olea europaea fruit oil (olive), tocopherol, cyclopentasiloxane, stearic acid, acrylates/c10 alkyl acrylate crosspolymer, methylparaben, propylparaben, citric acid, disodium EDTA, sodium hydroxide, DMDM hydantoin, BHT, fragrance, caramel, titanium dioxide, mica, dihydroxyacetone.

The first ingredient is water, which means this formula is mostly water. Based on the Brains' knowledge of lotions, it is about 80 percent water. Glycerin is the next most abundant ingredient, probably at about 5 percent. The next few ingredients are anywhere in the 1–3 percent range. Look at other skin lotions and you will find many of the same ingredients listed in the first line.

When you get to a "natural"-sounding ingredient like persea gratissima fruit extract, you've probably dropped below the magic 1 percent level. This is where manufacturers can start to make things look different. Generally speaking, natural ingredients are so expensive and so ineffective that only a trace amount is in there.

Most manufacturers like to put lots of these "feature" ingredients in the formula so they can show how their formula is different. The truth is the real functional work of the product is done primarily by the ingredients above this 1 percent line. The more abundant a material, the greater the effect it will have. Ingredients below the 1 percent line can provide benefits, but they are likely to be minimal compared to those that make up more than 1 percent.

Ingredients lists are included on your cosmetics to give you useful information about the products you use every day. They are put together following specific rules and if you know these rules, you can learn a lot about a product. The next time you're thinking of spending $25 on that upscale hair conditioner, compare the ingredients list to that of the $3 bottle. You might be surprised by the striking similarities. And if the chemicals are the same, you can bet they'll work similarly.

# REFERENCES

## CHAPTER 1:

(7) *Yes, studies have shown that coconut oil*    Ruetsch SB, Kamath YK, Rele AS, and Mohile RB. 2001. "Secondary ion mass spectrometric investigation of penetration of coconut and mineral oils into human hair fibers: relevance to hair damage." *J Cosmet Sci* 52: 169–84.

## CHAPTER 2:

(21) *Recently, there was a study done by researchers at the University of Utah*  Goates BM, Atkin JS, Wilding KG, Birch KG, Cottam MR, Bush SE, and Clayton DH. 2007. "An effective nonchemical treatment for head lice: a lot of hot air." *J Pediatr* (May) 150(5): 562–3.

## CHAPTER 3:

(33) *At any given moment, each hair follicle on your head*    Paus R and Cotsarelis G. 1999. "The biology of hair follicles." *New Engl J Med* 341(7): 491–7.

(34) *An article titled "Can dyeing your hair really give you cancer?"*  http://www.belfasttelegraph.co.uk/health/article2614806.ece

(35) *An article about hair dye and cancer*    Rollison DE, Helzlsouer KJ, and Pinney SM. 2006. "Personal hair dye use and cancer: a systematic literature review and evaluation of exposure assessment in studies published since 1992." *J Toxicol Environ Health B Crit Rev* (Sep-Oct) 9(5): 413–39.

(35) *For a more thorough summary of the cancer/hair color research*  http://jama/ama-assn.org/cgi/conent/abstract/293/20/2516

(43) *But according to the article*    Zimecki M. 2006. "The lunar cycle: effects on human and animal behavior and physiology." *Postepy Hig Med Dosw* 60: 1–7.

(44) *The second piece of the puzzle*   Fischer TW, Slominski A, Tobin DJ, and Paus R. 2008. "Melatonin and the hair follicle." *J Pineal Res* (Jan) 44(1): 1–15.

(46) *Should you attempt this on your own at home?*
http://www.hairfacts.com/tips/diyelectro/diyelectro.html

(46) *According to the FDA's Anthony Watson*   Segal M. 1996. "Hair today, gone tomorrow—removing unwanted hair." *FDA Consumer* (Sept).

# CHAPTER 4:

(54) *Retin-A is the brand name of a prescription drug called Tretinoin*
http://www.nlm.nih.gov/medlineplus/druginfo/meds/a682437.html

(57) *So, what about Imedeen?*  http://www.imedeen.us

(60) *Sound too good to be true? Check out the multiple clinical test results*
Bissett DL, et al. 2007. "Reduction in the appearance of facial hyperpigmentation by topical N-acetyl glucosamine." *J Cosmet Dermatol* (Mar) 6(1): 20–6.

(62) *Still confused about how to apply sunscreen?*   American Academy of Dermatology. http://www.aad.org/public/publications/pamphlets/sun_sunscreens.html

(64) *Yes, it's true, according to Anthony J. Mancini*   Focht DR, III, Spicer C, and Fairchok MP. 2002. "The efficacy of duct tape vs. cryotherapy in the treatment of verruca vulgaris (the common wart)." *Arch Pediatr Adolesc Med* (Oct) 156(10): 971–4.

(65) *No matter how a personal care product is marketed*   http://www.fda.gov/Cosmetics/GuidanceComplianceRegulatoryInformation/ucm074162.htm

(67) *Some compounds have been shown to have a UV-blocking effect when eaten*   Sies H and Stahl W. 2003. "Non-nutritive bioactive constituents of plants: lycopene, lutein and zeaxanthin." *Int J Vitam Nutr Res* (Mar) 73(2): 95–100.

(71) *According to company literature*   http://www.centerchem.com/PDFs/SYN-AKE%20Product%20Description.pdf

(74) *Let's start with an analysis of the components of the substance in question*
http://menshealth.about.com/cs/stds/a/about_semen.htm

(75) *Scientists originally thought that human saliva*   Oudhoff MJ, et al. 2009. "Structure-activity analysis of histatin, a potent wound healing peptide from human saliva: cyclization of histatin potentiates molar activity 1000-fold." *FASEB J* 23: 3928–35.

(76) *Poking your skin with a needle-studded roller*
http://www.derma-rollers.com/24/derma-roller-faqs

(76) *Amazing, isn't it? Here's how it works*    Fernandes D. 2005. "Minimally invasive percutaneous collagen induction." *Oral Maxillofacial Surg Clin N Am* 17: 51–63.

(78) *Finally, it's interesting to note that witch hazel is well-studied*    Wolff HH and Kieser M. 2007. "Hamamelis in children with skin disorders and skin injuries: results of an observational study." *Eur J Pediatr* (Sep) 166(9): 943–8.

(78) *Our story begins with squalene*    http://portalmarket.com/shark.html

(81) *From the Avon website*    http://www.avon.com

(82) *According to the American Society of Plastic Surgeons*    American Society of Plastic Surgeons. 2005. "Mesotherapy not proven as a safe alternative to liposuction." *Science Daily* (May). Retrieved August 26, 2010 from http://www.sciencedaily.com/releases/2005/05/050510193819.htm

(82) *Similarly, in a 2008 paper* Atiyeh BS, Ibrahim AE, Dibo SA. 2008. "Between scientific evidence, science fiction and lucrative business." *Aesth Plast Surg* 32: 842–9.

(84) *Checking the literature for specific research on the health effects of dryer sheets*    Juffres MR, Sampalli T, and Fox RA. 2005. "Physiologic and symptomatic responses to low-level substances in individuals with and without chemical sensitivities: a randomized controlled, blinded pilot booth study." *Environ Health Perspect* (Sep) 113(9): 1178–83.

(85) *Temporary skin rash, reddening or itchiness*    Mayo Clinic study. http://www.mayoclinic.org/allergic-diseases

(86) *Even though the FD&C Act defines*    "Is it a cosmetic, a drug, or both? (Or is it soap?)" http://www.fda.gov/Cosmetics/GuidanceComplianceRegulatoryInformation/ucm074201.htm

# CHAPTER 5:

(90) *Researchers at the University Hospital of Liege, Belgium*    Quatresooz P, Thirion L, Piérard-Franchimont C, and Piérard GE. 2006. "The riddle of genuine skin micro-relief and wrinkles." *Int J Cosmet Sci* (Dec) 28(6): 389–95.

(94) *Seven easy steps to popping your own pimples*    http://www.acne.org/pop.html

(95) *Rosacea is an inflammatory skin condition*   http://rosacea-support.org

(99) *Actually you* and *your friends might be right*   Zhai H and Maibach HI, eds. 2004. Dermatotoxicology, 6th ed. CRC Press: Boca Raton, Florida.

# CHAPTER 6:

(108) *Want another opinion? Paula Begoun, the Cosmetic Cop*
http://www.cosmeticscop.com

(118) *According to a team of psychologists*   http://www.cosmeticdesign-europe.com/formulation-science/make-up-really-does-work-scientists-claim

(118) *In their study, they found*   http://www.newscientist.com/article/dn8251-hormone-levels-predict-attractiveness-of-women.html

(120) *According to the company, the lip gloss*   http://www.omegatechlabs.com

(120) *While we are highly skeptical, there is some science backing up the concept behind this product*   Dr. Alan Hirsch. Smell and Taste Institute. http://www.smellandtaste.org

(121) *An interesting study*   Korichi R, Pelle-De-Queral D, Gazano G, and Aubert A. 2008. "Why women wear makeup: implication of psychological traits in makeup functions." *J Cosmet Sci* (Mar-Apr) 59: 127–37.

# CHAPTER 7:

(126) *Nearly all the popular brands of nail polish*   LoSasso GL, et al. 2002. "Neurocognitive sequelae of exposure to organic solvents and (meth)acrylates among nail-studio technicians." *Neuropsy Neuropsy Be* (Mar) 15(1): 44–55.

(129) *The idea that nail hardeners can help your nails grow longer*   American Academy of Dermatology. http://www.aad.org/media/background/factsheets/facts_nails.html

# CHAPTER 8:

(133) *However, flowery scents aren't for everyone*   Thyssen JP, et al. 2009. "Contact sensitization to fragrances in the general population: a Koch's approach may reveal the burden of disease." *Br J Dermatol* (Apr) 160(4): 729–35.

(134) *Perfume is wonderful*    International Flavors and Fragrance (IFF). http://www.iff.com

(137) *It is still debated among scientists whether pheromones have an effect* "SFSU study shows that synthetic pheromones in women's perfume increase intimate contact with men." http://www.sfsu.edu/~news/prsrelea/fy01/091.htm

(137) *In the study, four groups*    Hirsch A. "Special odor reduces perceived weight up to twelve pounds." http://www.smellandtaste.org/index.cfm?action=research.perceived

(140) *According to an article*    "Scent of tomorrow: scientists are going to unusual lengths to discover how your sense of smell influences the way you feel, eat, sleep, interact and reproduce." http://findarticles.com/p/articles/mi_m0NAH/is_4_34/ai_114783537

# CHAPTER 9:

(147) *Several new beauty gadgets on the market that do work*    Jesitus J. "Home laser use may boost derm visits." *Dermatology Times*, September 1, 2007.

(148) *The company can't say it, at least not anymore*    Laas M. "NAD suggests renovation of L'Oreal Nutritioniste claims from inside out." *The Rose Sheet*, August 1, 2007.

(151) *From a performance standpoint, no*    Consumer Reports, 2006. http://www.consumerreports.org/cro/home-garden/beauty-personal-care/cosmetics/wrinkle-creams-1-07/overview/0107_cream_ov_1.htm

(154) *While beauty companies do have great copywriters*    Cosmetics design-europe.com http://bit.ly/8njXgU

(155) *According to the FDA*    http://www.fda.gov/cosmetics/cosmeticlabelinglabelclaims/labelclaimsandexpirationdating/ucm2005203.htm

(156) *U.S. law defines cosmetics as*    "Is it a cosmetic, a drug, or both? (Or is it soap?)" http://www.fda.gov/Cosmetics/GuidanceComplianceRegulatoryInformation/ucm074201.htm

# CHAPTER 10:

(158) *We figured the article you mentioned was just a typical "scare" piece*    Macrae F. "Women absorb up to five pounds of damaging chemicals a year thanks to beauty products." http://www.dailymail.co.uk/health/article-462997/Women-absorb-5lbs-damaging-chemicals-year-thanks-beauty-products.html

(158) *The average woman absorbs 4lb, 6oz of chemicals*    "Trends in natural and organic cosmetics and toiletries." http://www.telegraph.co.uk/news/uknews/1555173/Body-absorbs-5lb-of-make-up-chemicals-a-year.html

(160) *The FDA believes that, at present, there*    http://www.fda.gov/cosmetics/productandingredientsafety/selectedcosmeticingredients/ucm128042.htm

(161) *So, where did the furor about parabens*    Darbre PD, Aljarrah A, Miller WR, Coldham NG, Sauer MJ, and Pope GS. 2004. "Concentrations of parabens in human breast tumours." *J Appl Toxicol* (Jan-Feb) 24(1): 5–13.

(166) *Experts agree that you should limit*    http://www.americanpregnancy.org

(169) *According to the Skin Medica website*    http://www.skinmedica.com

(171) *We couldn't find any medical references*    "Antiperspirant safety." http://www.unilever.com/brands/hygieneandwelbeing/antiperspirant_safety/?WT.LHNAV=Antiperspirant_safety

(173) *The FDA has reported that the parasite cryptosporidium*    "FDA warns consumers about the risk of cryptosporidium illness from Baby's Bliss gripe water," September 20, 2007. http://www.fda.gov/NewsEvents/Newsroom/PressAnnouncements/2007/ucm108990.htm

# INDEX